About DEATH
From a Cancer Doctor's Perspective

By
James W. Forsythe, M.D., H.M.D.

About Death From a Cancer Doctor's Perspective

Century Wellness Publishing

Copyright © 2013, By James W. Forsythe, M.D., H.M.D.

All Rights Reserved, including the right of
Reproduction in whole or in part in any form.

Forsythe, James W. M.D., H.M.D.
Book Design: Patty Atcheson Melton

1. Health 2. Death

NOTICE: The author of this book and accompanying programs used his best efforts to prepare this publication. The author and publisher make no representation or warranties with respect to the accuracy, applicability, or completeness of the contents in this book. The author disclaims any warranties (express or implied), as to the merchantability, or fitness of the text herein for any particular purpose. The author and publisher shall in no event be held liable for any loss or other damages. Any person diagnosed with a terminal illness or with a terminal injury, and/or relatives, friends and acquaintances of such individuals, should visit a certified, licensed physician or mental health professional; only such professionals are qualified and licensed to make a medical diagnosis and/or to prescribe medications or treatment regimens.

This book contains material protected under International and Federal Copyright Laws and Treaties. Any unauthorized reprint or use of this material is prohibited, under civil and federal and governmental penalties.

ISBN: 978-0-9897636-1-5

Dedication

To "death" as well as to "life," the universal forces of change.

"No one wants to die. Even people who want to get to heaven don't want to die to get there. And yet death is the destination we all share. No one has ever escaped it, and that is as it should be, because death is very likely the single best invention of life. It's life's change agent. It clears out the old, and makes way for the new."

-**Steve Jobs**

Contents

Foreword
7

Chapter 1: Face Your Doom
9

Chapter 2: Death "Becomes You"
14

Chapter 3: Short-Term Victories Against Death
18

Chapter 4: Acknowledge Fear
22

Chapter 5: My Battle Against Death Intensified
30

Chapter 6: Many Health Issues Rival Cancer
36

Chapter 7: Death Defined
48

Chapter 8: Certifying Death
57

Chapter 9: The Good, the Bad and the Ugly
64

Chapter 10: Modern Communication Worsens Issues
74

Chapter 11: Question: What Happens When we Die?
78

Chapter 12: The Five Stages of Grief
90

Chapter 13: Death-Related Issues Abound
108

Chapter 14: Technology Issues
127

Chapter 15: Apparent "Life After Death"
131
Chapter 16: Religion and Philosophy Enter the Equation
149
Chapter 17: "Spooky" Belief Systems
170
Chapter 18: Death-Defying Acts Abound
177
Chapter 19: Humanity's Quest for Massive Death
182
Chapter 20: Death by Execution
195
Chapter 21: Death Customs
211
Chapter 22: Burning Bodies
219
Chapter 23: Funeral Rituals
224
Chapter 24: Death in Modern and Historical Cultures
236
Chapter 25: Meet the "Grim Reaper"
250
Chapter 26: My Own Death
258
About the Author
266

Foreword

Since you first picked up this book, several people have died at various places worldwide. That's what happens every second—numerous individuals depart from this earthly life.

Amazingly, I had my own brush with the black-caped Grim Reaper just one day after I finished writing the initial draft of this book.

Let me start from the beginning of this tale so that you will clearly understand.

During the spring of 2013 I finally caved in to the many requests from my patients, friends and associates worldwide who had asked me to write this book, in the wake of my many other successful publications. Collectively and individually, these people had asked me to give the urgent advice found on the pages that follow.

Anyway, from that point forward I spent nearly five months thinking about, researching and writing the initial manuscript, working in conjunction with my professional advisors.

Then, suddenly during the second week of August that year I felt a severe pain in my chest and a shortness of breath.

In a flash that day a life-threatening heart situation forced me to go into action to save myself. My adopted daughter played an integral role in helping to save me. I told her: "This is serious. I'm not joking. I'm going to need your help. Honey, please do as I say."

At the time we were at Lake Tahoe, a one-hour drive from my Reno home. I promptly did what most physicians recommend that people do to potentially save themselves in such situations—I took two aspirins to thin my blood. I also took nitroglycerin heart medicine, retrieved from my medical bag.

Several weeks later following a grim diagnosis my cardiologist recommended an immediate stent procedure due to excessive plaque within the artery leading into my heart. Although such procedures are relatively common in the United States, as a doctor I know full well that a chance of sudden death exists while a stent is inserted into the blood stream.

Right before my loving, dutiful and intelligent wife Earlene took me to the hospital for this procedure I gave her what many people might consider a dying request: "Please promise that if I die, you'll make sure that my book about death is published and sold worldwide. What the book teaches is critical for people to know."

Of course, I obviously survived. In the process my doctors discovered that I had been much closer to potential death than any of us had initially realized. Excessive plaque had blocked more than 90 percent of the natural blood flow to my heart. The insertion of a stent into the main artery enabled life-giving blood to efficiently pump into the organ.

Needless to say, following my recovery I made the publication of this book a top priority. Perhaps more than ever I felt a burning need to repeat that age-old saying: "Seeing an old man die is like watching a library burn."

So, remember, I literally made the publication of this book my "dying request."

It's that important. As you might imagine, I pray that you, your family or loved one learn the vital details that you need to know about death in the pages that follow.

-James W. Forsythe, M.D., H.M.D.

Chapter 1

Face Your Doom

Tales of human sacrifice, death, violence, and murder have all permeated literature and poetry for thousands of years.

Today's rapid-fire Information Super-highway, from around-the-clock cable TV to online book distribution and video games, has bombarded the public mindset with death.

Long after the iconic bard William Shakespeare penned such classics as the romantic, tragic suicides of "Romeo & Juliet" the topic of death permeates virtually every significant aspect of our culture.

A vast array of media ranging from the Beatles' hit song "Help" in the 1960s about human sacrifice to classic novels by horror writer Stephen King are widely accepted throughout society.

Indeed, there's no escaping the fact that death prevails as a dominant daily topic throughout society. This psychological bombardment often starts shortly after we awaken each morning to hear about the latest celebrity deaths on the morning news. The onslaught of death information usually continues late at night, when many of us finally begin bedtime after watching the latest hot cable TV show about murder.

Yes, you are going to die someday.

There will be no escape.

You'll be murdered, succumb to injuries from an accident, pass away from natural causes, starve or get wiped out in a disaster such as drowning or wounds from an earthquake or tornado.

Right from the start here, you can consider me as perhaps one of the world's premiere experts on the topic of death.

You see, I've personally known 12,000 people who have died.

I had worked to cure these individuals of cancer when serving as their medical doctor.

While I thought that I was learning how to live, I have been learning how to die.
- Leonardo da Vinci

Today, I'm known worldwide as a unique, extremely rare "cancer doctor," one of only a handful of integrative medical oncologists in the United States.

Now on the verge of marking my 50th year as a practicing doctor, as a physician I now have one of the highest cancer "cure" rates in North America and the entire world.

Until the mid-1990s, about 97 percent of my Stage IV cancer patients died from their disease.

The death rates of such patients visiting my clinic have changed markedly since I incorporated natural treatments into my practice beginning in the late 1990s. Now, on average from 45 percent to 85 percent of my Stage IV cancer patients are "cured."

Yet I can guarantee with 100 percent certainty that virtually all of those who experienced the loss of their cancer will someday die of still-to-be-determined causes.

Life is hard. Then you die. Then they throw dirt in your face. Then the worms eat you. Be grateful it happens in that order.
- David Gerrold

Needless to say, at least as of the time this book was initially published, I remained what some people hailed as one of the world's premiere living experts on the subject of death.

James W. Forsythe, M.D., H.M.D.

At least judging by published accounts, I've personally known more people who have died than the notorious "Angel of Death," physician Joseph Mengele ~ the Nazi torturer and killer of thousands of Jews in World War II concentration camps.

Like this or not, I've even personally known far more people who have died than the late Doctor Jacob "Jack" Kevorkian, a pathologist heralded as "Doctor Death" due to his willingness to assist 130 terminally or chronically ill people to commit suicide.

At the onset here, I feel a need to proclaim that my distinction of personally knowing countless people who have died should never be considered as a "badge of honor."

Far more important, my extensive experience interacting with dying people and their families affords me an opportunity to teach you here about the inescapable topic of dying.

Death most resembles a prophet who is without honor in his own land or a poet who is a stranger among his people.
- **Khalil Gibran**

One of the world's premiere, best-known experts on this topic was Elisabeth Kübler-Ross, author of the 1969 bestseller, "On Death and Dying." The publication followed her many years of intense initial research as a pioneer in the death process.

Kübler-Ross earned worldwide fame at a time while I served as a doctor in the Vietnam War, personally conducting hundreds of autopsies on U.S. soldiers and working with other American Army medical experts in treating our wounded comrades.

In her first major book, Kübler-Ross identified and chronicled what she heralded as the "five" stages of grief—denial, anger, bargaining, depression and acceptance.

Early in my career I used this Swiss-American psychiatrist's essential findings as a basis for my own discoveries on the death and dying process.

My findings as chronicled in subsequent chapters of this book

About Death

likely will spark controversy and intense public discussion, while hopefully serving as critically helpful to people facing imminent death.

Certainly, there have been numerous books and articles published about death since Kübler-Ross died at age 78 in 2004, after stating that she was ready for death, following a series of debilitating strokes.

I have never killed a man. But I have read many obituaries with great pleasure.
*~ **Clarence Darrow***

In all likelihood at this very moment, you're still ensconced in denial—refusing to acknowledge your own pending death, despite my strident declaration earlier on the first page that "you will die."

Without delay, you'll soon learn the mysterious and complex reasons why right now you're still likely refusing to accept this irrefutable fact.

Just as important, why will you die? Why will everyone that you know now, or will ever know in the future, suffer a similar fate?

How will you grieve your own pending death? How can you cope with the future deaths of your loved ones, even if you're already experienced at such intense grief?

Learn why you fantasize about escaping death. What will you think during your final moments? How will you mentally and physically fight to remain alive, despite the inevitable? When and will you intrinsically know that "the time" has arrived, perhaps an opportunity for your final surrender?

I've told my children that when I die, to release balloons in the sky to celebrate when I graduated. For me, death is a graduation.
*- **Elisabeth Kübler-Ross***

James W. Forsythe, M.D., H.M.D.

Like many people, perhaps you've seen the countless daily obituaries, stating that the deceased "fought a courageous battle" against the disease or affliction that killed them.

Soon, you'll learn why we fight to remain alive and why such struggles are indeed good and righteous.

Yet many of us will also discover what for some of us shall become the inevitable need to open up our bodies, hearts and minds in full acceptance of Mother Nature's 100-percent guarantee—certain, unavoidable death.

In all likelihood, on the day after you die the world will keep turning and billions of other people will continue going about their daily lives—seemingly as if you were "unimportant." When that happens, almost all of them will continue denying their own impending deaths.

Since as the old saying goes "life is for the living," for the time being you can benefit by embracing the lessons that I'm about to give.

I didn't attend the funeral, but I sent a nice letter saying I approved of it.
-Mark Twain

Chapter 2

Death "Becomes You"

As a 12-year-old child in Detroit long before I became a doctor, I arrived home from school one day and immediately found my aunt dead on the living room floor.

To this day I vividly recall the curdling cries of my uncle. He wept non-stop the next 24 hours as the love of his life's death of natural causes ravaged his psyche.

Whether expected or shockingly sudden, death almost always mortifies and ravages the spirits and minds of those of us who remain alive. Severe depression often results.

Dealing directly with death can also prove harrowing for aspiring medical professionals. I vividly recall some of my classmates becoming nauseous and extremely ill as we dissected cadavers in medical school in San Francisco in the early 1960s.

Facing the issue of death becomes unavoidable for doctors, particularly in combat situations. Within a few months after I became close friends with a nurse, Lt. Sharon Ann Lane, during my 1969 tour of duty in Vietnam, she suffered mortal shrapnel wounds during a rocket attack. Lane became the first female U.S. soldier killed in combat in Vietnam; four other American women had previously died during that war from illness or aircraft crashes.

Soon after the 25-year-old Lane's death on June 8, 1969, at the 312th Evacuation Hospital, I performed the autopsy on her as required by military regulations. This emerged as one of the first of what would eventually become many thousands of deaths of persons that I had personally known.

James W. Forsythe, M.D., H.M.D.

The fear of death follows from the fear of life. A man who lives fully is prepared to die at any time.

- Mark Twain

During my one-year tour in Vietnam I feared for my life in several near-death situations. I ran for cover during an enemy attack at our base, and soon fortified my barracks living quarters bed with sandbags for added protection from future attacks.

Soon afterward like countless other U.S. soldiers during the war I feared for my life amid an unexpected traumatic situation. As one of more than a dozen Army personnel on a helicopter, I expected the worst as we crash landed on the beach of a small island off the South Vietnam coast in the South China Sea.

Each of us escaped serious injury before spending the night on the beach, unsure of whether the enemy might attack at any moment. Thankfully a rescue craft arrived early the next day to take us back to the South Vietnam mainland.

Shortly after my discharge from the military and upon re-entering to military life, I decided to become an oncologist. At the time the specialization for treating cancer was considered unique.

During that era many medical specialties emerged. Although viewed as unique at the time, today lots of these practices are considered rather commonplace As a new cancer specialist starting in the early 1970s, I anticipated that over the course years I would deal with many deaths. Yet I had no idea that death would suddenly and unexpectedly cause severe anguish and hardship within my family.

A friend who dies, it's something of you who dies.

-Gustave Flaubert

Several few years after returning from the war and entering private practice, I moved from the San Francisco Bay Area to

About Death

become partners with a physician in Reno, Nevada. I eventually started my own oncology practice, and fell in love with Earlene, an attractive and brilliant woman who would later become my wife.

As my relationship with Earlene solidified, her ex-husband was decapitated during a horrific highway accident. The mental and physical trauma impacted our entire immediate family as we strived to cope with the unexpected sudden shock.

A so-called "double whammy" hit in the late 1970s when the husband of Earlene's sister, Val, was killed in a car accident on an isolated Nevada highway. Several of the couple's children were critically injured in the wreck, while Val escaped extreme physical trauma.

Immediately upon learning of the tragedy I rushed to the hospital to assist in the children's medical care. I assisted in implementing various medical procedures and administered natural substances intended to accelerate their recoveries.

During that decade I began to personally witness and experience death on an industrial scale. As stated earlier, nearly a half century ago the "cure" or "recovery" rates were extremely low among Stage IV cancer patients receiving standard-medical treatments.

Those who have the strength and the love to sit with a dying patient in the silence that goes beyond words will know that this moment is neither frightening nor painful, but a peaceful cessation of the functioning of the body.

-Elisabeth Kübler-Ross

During the early 1970s the primary industry-dictated protocol among standard-medicine oncologists treating such patients was essentially the same then as it is today. This meant killing much of the body with poisonous chemo or radiation in attempts to eradicate cancer.

James W. Forsythe, M.D., H.M.D.

Mirroring the average results of oncologists nationwide during that period, a whopping 97 out every 100 of my Stage IV cancer patients died in the 1970s and 1980s.

Rather than become emotionally cold or "heartless" in dealing with these people, I deeply cared for each of them while increasingly thinking "there has to be a better way."

Instead of immediately perceiving each patient as "doomed" upon reaching a diagnosis, I wholeheartedly strived to "save" or "cure" each and every person.

In the process while always remaining highly professional, I became close friends with or emotionally bonded with many of them.

Remember, all this happened several decades before my clinic's overall "cure" rates skyrocketed upward—generating some of the nation's highest Stage IV cancer recovery rates now during the 21st Century.

Dying is easy; it's living that scares me to death.
-Annie Lennox

Chapter 3
Short-Term Victories Against Death

Boosted by harmless natural medicines now during the 21st Century, the irrefutable results of my clinic's cancer recovery rates continue generating extreme jealousy and anger among many standard-medicine oncologists.

For me as a medical professional during the late 1970s and early 1980s, long before incorporating natural treatments into my practice, the death process became increasingly important in my personal life and in my work.

Throughout that era I remained an officer in the Army National Guard. While riding as a passenger in a military plane from the Pacific Northwest toward Reno, the aircraft experienced severe engine problems.

Passengers were told to prepare for a horrific potential outcome as we made the final approach of several hundred miles toward our Northwest Nevada home.

I securely fastened my safety belt as natural fears seized my psyche. Although a highly educated physician well aware by that point that "death is a natural end of life," survival became my top priority.

The survival instinct remains just as natural and predictable as the final and inescapable "Grim Reaper." Lucky for me and for my fellow passengers our plane soon made a safe landing.

Years later, extreme engine trouble in a private airplane

James W. Forsythe, M.D., H.M.D.

forced Earlene and I to fear for our lives. As we rode in the aircraft from Davis, California, for several hundred miles back to Reno we wondered whether death would suddenly arrive.

A dying man needs to die as a sleepy man needs to sleep, and there comes a time when it is wrong, as well as useless, to resist.
-Stewart Alsop

Following my tenth anniversary as a doctor, in the late 1970s I began teaching a course on dying at the University of Nevada Medical School.

Much of my teaching hinged on the groundbreaking research and reports of Elisabeth Kübler-Ross—critical and basic issues ranging from denial to acceptance.

More than their predecessors did when I taught the course, medical students now amid the 21st Century need to learn how to address the issue of death.

Modern patients have far greater and faster access to vital medical information than such people endured as recently as the last half of the 1900s.

A deep, intense fear of death is now motivating cancer patients and their relatives or friends to demand immediate answers.

Common questions range from "how long do I have?" to "how painful will this be," and of course the understandable "what are my chances for a cure?"

As a rare integrative medical oncologist with far more experience dealing with death than the vast majority of currently practicing doctors, I have developed genuine, heartfelt and sincere ways of dealing directly with such inquiries.

Death will be a great relief. No more interviews.
- Katherine Hepburn

About Death

In all honesty, when dealing with my patients and staff I have managed to approach and to deal with death in a highly professional manner.

Yet a deep need for openness when teaching people about the emotional and physical intricacies of this unavoidable process—death—has motivated me to reveal here what many patients and staffers have never known until now.

Although fully sane and retaining full control of my mental capacities, on many occasions I have wept for my dying or dead patients.

When alone in my office or while driving in my car, sometimes while waiting at intersections at traffic lights, intense grief occasionally overwhelms my psyche.

I grieve for my patients, whom I love or care for deeply on a spiritual and emotional level. Often I grieve for their families as well. My heart goes out to the loss that the survivors have sustained, and for the hardships the disease has forced them to endure.

Sometimes rivers of tears stream down my cheeks and cascade onto my shirt. On other occasions my eyes become wet and red, the tears refusing to reveal themselves.

Man always dies before he is fully born.
                                                    - **Erich Fromm**

Never a crier by nature, I'm a strong-willed man. Without such mental fortitude I never would have been able to defy the dictates of the standard-medicine community, developing new natural remedies regimen that have substantially improved my clinic's "cure" rates.

Certainly, for a doctor to truly care, he or she needs to be "human." For me, this means genuinely caring emotionally and professionally for each and every one of my patients. Throughout my career, many times I have witnessed doctors at other hospitals or clinics interacting with patients as if those individuals were mere "rats on a treadmill."

Perhaps in many instances some standard-medicine oncologists who administer only deadly chemo and radiation take an arms-length approach with patients. This way perhaps at least in part these doctors can strive to avoid becoming emotionally attached.

Ultimately, of course—unlike most doctors—all the various consequences and emotions involving death involve patients, their families and friends.

Meantime, as a physician holding the extremely rare designation of "integrative medical oncologist," like most other doctors with each patient I strive to give the best most effective treatment possible—with the objective of generating ideal results.

From my rotting body flowers shall grow and I am in them and that is eternity.
-Edvard Munch

Chapter 4

Acknowledge Fear

Virtually all of us carry this unspoken fear.

Either from pluralistic ignorance or perhaps basic denial, we all know that someday we'll personally experience the death and dying process.

Yet rarely is this topic discussed, as noted by Kübler-Ross in her various groundbreaking books and articles.

Based on what I've seen and experienced in my personal and professional lives, we all experience various degrees of emotions and reactions when death grabs those we know and love. Usually these episodes involve the sudden or unexpected demise of loved ones or acquaintances, until dying ourselves.

Like just about every person my age, I have been forced to cope with many deaths throughout my personal life—beginning from early childhood.

Other than the separation or "death" of my parents relationship when I was 2 ½ years old, some of the many instances included the fear of my own potential death when hit by a car at age 4, plus the mysterious unsolved death of my maternal grandmother.

The death of a top athlete that I knew as a teen, knowing someone killed by lightening and the suicide death of my best high school friend's father added to my experiences. Then, my best friend in college, John, killed himself.

A man who won't die for something is not fit to live.
                                        -Rev. Dr. Martin Luther King Jr.

James W. Forsythe, M.D., H.M.D.

Yes, virtually all of us—particularly people who have survived at least into our mid-20s and beyond—have had multiple encounters with or come close to others who died.

Predictably, the personal interaction with the dying process multiplies many-fold among people who become doctors or who enter various areas of the medical profession.

While attending medical school in San Francisco, one of my close friends—a classmate—died of cancer.

One of my earliest direct experiences with death as a healthcare professional involved a woman who died in childbirth while I attended medical school.

These episodes occurred during the so-called "hippy generation" while I studied and worked in San Francisco. At the time this famed city by the bay served as a magnet for young people within the anti-war generation, many of them embracing what Timothy Leary called the "tune-in, turn-on, drop-out" philosophy.

At the height of this social revolution I worked as a physician at a drug clinic in San Francisco's famed Haight-Ashbury district where countless hippies congregated.

During 1968, the year before my Army tour of duty in Vietnam, I treated numerous people who died from overdoses after they ingested heroin, psychedelic drugs, barbiturates, Quaaludes or speed.

Earlier in 1968 while on assignment for the military on the East Coast, while traveling by car through Washington, D.C., my family got surrounded by deadly riots that erupted nationwide following the assassination of the Rev. Dr. Martin Luther King Jr.
The dead cannot cry out for justice. It is a duty of the living to do so for them.
- Lois McMaster Bujold

One of my close friends has called me a "real-live version of the iconic fictional movie character Forrest Gump—a lucky guy

About Death

who made amazing business or personal discoveries—in my case supposedly "developing a cure for cancer."

Of course, such a statement is a wild, off-the-mark exaggeration for I have not come close to eliminating the disease—although my average Stage IV cancer patients as an overall group experience far better outcomes than the nationwide average.

Even so, I've got to admit that at least in some ways my life seems to have mirrored the story of Gump, who stumbles upon many of the most traumatic events of the 1960s.

For instance, in 1963 while attending medical school I was among the last physicians to treat the famed Gen. Douglas MacArthur before he died in his early 80s.

Later, while I served as a pathologist briefly at Womack Army Medical Hospital at Fort Bragg in North Carolina, I investigated heat-related deaths in which meningitis was listed as a contributing factor.

My personal interaction with the death process seemed to accelerate from that point. In 1970, following my Vietnam tour both parents of one of my friends died of lung cancer. Amid this period, although outwardly behaving as professional, my heart shattered when treating several youngsters who died at a children's hospital.

Death is a very dull, dreary affair, and my advice to you is to have nothing whatsoever to do with it.
- W. Somerset Maugham

Determined to support my first wife and young children during that period, I simultaneously worked numerous doctor duties at various hospitals and clinics.

My work in the Emergency Room at Saint Francis Memorial Hospital in San Francisco motivated me to strive to save trauma victims—many who eventually died.

James W. Forsythe, M.D., H.M.D.

My first wife and I divorced during that period, when my medical work duties forced me to remain away from home for extended periods. At that point, well before meeting my current wife, Earlene—the love of my life—I continued working at Saint Francis.

During 1973 and 1974, I treated many patients for leukemia, various other diseases and for what eventually became the first known cases of AIDS—which physicians later identified in the late 1970s and early 1980s.

My professional interaction with death soon accelerated at a rapid rate, until finally subsiding somewhat when I started integrating remedies into the treatments of my cancer patients beginning in the late 1990s.

Millions long for immortality who don't know what to do with themselves on a rainy Sunday afternoon.
-Susan Ertz

The father of my girlfriend, Genevieve, died from cancer in 1974. Soon afterward, the course of my life changed markedly when she and I traveled together to Reno from San Francisco for his funeral and to handle estate matters.

At that juncture I needed to do something to boost my income while helping Genevieve financially and also supporting my ex-wife and children.

So, during my brief stay in Northwest Nevada with her, I seized that opportunity to arrange a job interview with a cancer-treatment doctor in Reno.

Because that physician was the only oncologist in Northern Nevada at the time his cancer patient totals steadily increased in that area, and his business surged.

Faced with perhaps more business than he could personally handle, the doctor brought me in as a physician at his clinic and eventually as a partner with the long-term agreement of me eventually assuming ownership and operation of the practice.

Soon afterward, the shortage of cancer specialists in Reno motivated me to become the chief of oncology simultaneously in that region's two largest medical facilities at the time—Washoe Medical Hospital, later called Renown, and also Saint Mary's Hospital.

Pale death beats equally at the poor man's gate and at the palaces of kings.

-**Horace**

Following my breakup with Genevieve, my romantic relationship launched with Earlene—the drop-dead attractive and brilliant nurse in Reno, whom I eventually married. All along, my professional work pace accelerated at breakneck speed.

Still as the only experienced oncologist in an entire widespread region of the United States, the Northwest Nevada area, I seemingly worked around-the-clock in an effort to help as many patients as I could.

For much of that time I lacked any nurses on my staff, also without similar professionals to work late-night or early morning shifts.

This left me with no other option than to personally administer chemotherapy substances or various medicines. I did all that work all by myself. The process chewed up many hours of my daily work time, periods when I could have been seeing additional patients who desperately needed my help.

My so-called "Forrest Gump experiences" soon blasted into overdrive. During the 1950s, the U.S. government had conducted above-ground nuclear bomb tests in the Nevada desert. Countless people who came into contact with nuclear fallout radiation spread by the experiments gradually started getting cancer during subsequent decades.

Thousands of people who had lived downwind from the

James W. Forsythe, M.D., H.M.D.

explosions during the 1950s and early 1960s streamed to my office beginning in the late 1970s. At the time, mandatory criteria or protocol stipulated that I administer poisonous and often-deadly chemo and/or radiation treatments to all Stage IV cancer patients.

It is possible to provide security against other ills, but as far as death is concerned, we men live in a city without walls.

- Epicurus

Suddenly, I found myself engulfed in a situation where I had personally become involved in death on an "industrial scale."

In a sense I had became more personally involved with people in the process of dying than Alexander the Great, U.S. Gen. George Patton, Napoleon Bonaparte, Stalin, Lenin and Mao Tse Tung.

These world-famous military leaders or revolutionaries orchestrated the deaths of countless millions of people in wars or government overthrows. For the most part, these infamous or widely known world figures did not personally know the warriors who had died for them, or the many victims of their slaughter.

By contrast, I have personally known and loved in a spiritual or professional way virtually every one of the more than 12,000 individuals who have died while under my care—an average of 300 people yearly, continuously over a 40-year period.

Over time, my patient-death total grew to more than four times the total number of Americans killed in the entire Spanish-American War. The U.S. death toll during that international conflict reached 2,910 according to government data.

Although like any doctor "never proud" of the combined death count of my patients, many people become surprised to learn that I have personally treated: Nearly five times more people who eventually died than the 2,260 U.S. Army soldiers killed in the War of 1812; more than eight times the total 1,500 people who perished in the 1912 sinking of the RMS Titanic; and nearly four times the estimated 3,155 Union Army soldiers who perished in the Battle of

About Death

Gettysburg in July 1863 during the American Civil war.

"How have you coped with this, doctor?" some patients might ask me, those who know the truth. "What is your secret to remaining mentally sharp and as good as ever?"

As you'll soon discover, the many reasons for this are specific yet varied.

Since the day of my birth, my death began its walk. It is walking toward me, without hurrying.
- Jean Cocteau

Amazingly, judging by my own recollection, I was nearly among 70 people killed by an airplane crash early on Monday morning of January 20, 1985.

For me the previous night had been typical and rather ordinary. I had worked through the midnight hour assisting critically ill and dying patients at the Reno area's two primary hospitals.

Weary, tired as usual and eager to awaken before sunrise later that morning—intending to catch a few hours sleep, I drove quietly through empty streets toward my home in an area that at the time was south of the Reno city limits.

I cruised southbound on South Virginia Street, also known at the time as U.S. Highway 395. Within blocks of my destination, at 1:04 a.m. Pacific Standard Time, I heard a tremendous bang coming from somewhere behind me—and noticed a brief flash of light in my rear-view mirror.

It wasn't until the following morning that I learned that the bang and flash had been from the crash of Galaxy Airlines Flight 203. All but one of the 71 people on board perished in the fiery crash on the highway. Without any doubt whatsoever, I realized that if I had been driving just a tiny bit slower the jetliner would have crashed onto me.

"Thank you, God, for saving me," I thought, realizing that I had just escaped almost certain death. "Lord, you must have spared me for a good reason, part of your grand plan. Let me be worthy, perhaps by finding a way to save far more people from cancer."

Some people are so afraid to die that they never begin to live.
-**Henry Van Dyke**

Chapter

5

My Battle Against Death Intensified

Every month from around the world, streams of patients seeking treatment for cancer and other ailments travel to my Reno clinic.

Rather than serving as a facility for death on an "industrial scale" as its predecessor had, my current facility offers a genuine new chance at healthy life for most patients.

As stated earlier, thanks largely to the natural remedies that I now provide as one of only a handful of integrative medical oncologists in the United States, the Stage IV cancer survival or "cure" rates at my facility is much higher than at most other clinics.

The positive word of mouth has spread, the indisputable fact that I'm in the "life" business rather than in the "death industry."

Perhaps my many successful books on various medical topics ranging from the Forsythe Anti-Cancer Diet to Natural Pain Cures have played a formidable role in boosting my professional reputation.

Certainly positive word-of-mouth has also emerged as a major factor, probably at least partly because people are increasingly angry with the mainstream medical industry that pushes highly poisonous chemotherapy. People are demanding "a better way."

With this in mind the personal experiences, symptoms and prognosis of each individual patient remains of utmost importance.

'Tis very certain the desire of life prolongs it.
                                                    -Lord Byron

James W. Forsythe, M.D., H.M.D.

My death-related responsibilities and experiences spread to new realms during my first few decades in Reno.

While continuing my own practice and overseeing oncology services at two hospitals, I became the director of hospice care for Hearthstone of Northern Nevada, a major extended care facility.

As if these many responsibilities weren't already enough, I still felt a need to do more to help as many people as possible.

Increasingly motivated to help more many families of people with cancer, I served as a founding board member of the Ronald McDonald House Charities Reno facility—designed to help the well being and health of children.

Even more responsibilities evolved when I also simultaneously became the director of hospice care at several Reno nursing homes.

Rather than rip at my psyche, these added responsibilities helped give me a greater sense of self-fulfillment. Yet an inner-sense within my spirit kept telling me that perhaps I could be doing much more.

Perhaps I could do my utmost to "cure" cancer, at least in a sense that perhaps I might be able to find a way to put far more cancers in remission among my many patients.

The timing of death, like the ending of a story, gives a changed meaning to what preceded it.

- Mary Catherine Bateman

Along my pathway to completely transforming my business and getting additional formal medical education in hopes of "finding a better way," the deaths of my patients and several of my close friends steadily increased my motivation.

Unbendingly patriotic and wanting to continually serve our country to the best of my ability, into the late 1990s I continued to

About Death

serve as an officer in the U.S. Army National Guard.

As if my regular professional experiences with death weren't already enough, I got saddled with the responsibility of investigating as a pathologist the deaths of several soldiers as they attended summer camp training in Death Valley.

Autopsies and research conducted under my command led me to conclude that the perished soldiers died from heat exposure

My medical expertise and extensive knowledge of the death process also left me with no other option than to investigate the death of one of my friends. My findings concluded that this man died of natural causes, likely a massive heart attack, while having sex with a woman other than his wife in a motel room.

Meanwhile, several people whom I had first met when they were healthy subsequently got cancer and eventually died. In numerous instances some of these individuals perished despite my best efforts, at the time my hands essentially cuffed together by the mainstream medical industry's protocol requiring that only chemo and/or radiation are permissible treatments for certain advanced cancers.

The idea is to die young as late as possible.
-Ashley Montagu

In the late 1990s I began intensive studies to earn a doctorate degree in natural medicine, unwilling to accept the demented dictates of the misguided mainstream medical industry.

By that point I needed to face the fact that the mainstream medical industry is corrupt or inept—or perhaps even both. Hailed as a "maverick" by some of my associates and even as a "egotistical tyrant" by my misguided adversaries, I refused to accept the notion that poisons would eventually save people.

As a comparison, these days as an overall society we look back in revulsion and at least some degree of perplexity at the era from the 1500s well into the 1800s. Many people today admit to feeling emotionally stunned upon learning when doctors and patients were convinced that "bleeding treatments" would remove disease from the bodies of ill or injured people.

To the contrary, of course, thanks to so-called modern medicine we know that intentionally cutting and bleeding patients was tantamount to quackery. Perhaps more patients died from those reckless treatments than from the underlying diseases.

Ironically, probably jealous of my clinic's high-cure rates, lots of today's standard-medicine oncologists that administer the most deadly chemo possible and other mainstream doctors insist on referring to me as a "quack."

Who knows for sure? Maybe those doctors who insist on criticizing me are jealous, or perhaps some of them fully believe all of the hogwash taught to them in medical school that dictates "chemotherapy is the only way to go."

Indeed, shouldn't the tide of criticism be turned in the direction of my harshest critics within the medical industry rather than toward me? Maybe the oncologists who insist on administering only highly poisonous chemo in all instances of severe cancer should be considered "quacks." This seems logical. After all, only a fool would dare give an extreme poison to a every person with advanced cancer, never giving those individuals the option of potentially effective non-toxic and natural remedies. Yet that is exactly what mainstream oncologists insist on doing.

All our knowledge merely helps us to die a more painful death than animals who know nothing.
-Maurice Maeterlinck

Besides striving to improve a patient's quality of life, standard-medicine or "allopathic" physicians must follow dictates mandated by the misguided U.S. Food and Drug Administration—commonly known as the FDA—and rules solidified by their peers.

Rather than remain on that deadly treadmill and willingly to continue participating in that failed system, I took a step forward in seeking a new course of action.

This undoubtedly struck the vast majority of my peers as rebellious, particularly as I became a licensed homeopath while simultaneously maintaining my longtime standard allopathic license.

My choices irked lots of traditional oncologists nationwide and around the globe. They complained that I had started proclaiming that Homeopathy serves as a pathway to potential life for Stage IV cancer patients rather than almost-certain death.

"People are fed up with false propaganda from the FDA," I started to say. "I choose to show such patients a potential pathway toward a greater probability of remaining alive—rather than the route to almost certain death embraced by allopathic medicine."

To be idle is a short road to death and to be diligent is a way of life. Foolish people are idle; wise people are diligent.
-Buddha

All along I also became increasingly determined to teach people about the process of death and dying. Everyone deserves the truth about this critical topic, particularly those observing the death process as friends and relatives of the terminally ill, or people in the process of dying from various illnesses.

Sadly, I have witnessed many hundreds or perhaps even thousands of instances where allopathic physicians avoid discussing death the topic with terminal patients and their families. Worsening matters, huge numbers of doctors also fail to direct dying patients toward helpful services or facilities such as hospices.

These shameless and reckless oversights likely will accelerate at a rapid rate in the near future unless the medical industry heeds the advice I'm about to give.

A huge percentage of the U.S. population is entering their senior years at a record rate. As of the 2013, every day a mind-numbing 8,000 American citizens were reaching age 65, according to the American Association of Retired Persons or AARP.

As dictated by the aging process, a huge variety of deadly ailments gradually afflict elderly individuals. Besides cancer, the steadily growing tide of fatal diseases impacting seniors range from heart problems to Alzheimer's Disease and many other ailments.

I'm not afraid of dying. I just don't want to be there when it happens.
-Woody Allen

Chapter 6
Many Health Issues Rival Cancer

Today, numerous famous charitable organizations from the American Heart Association to the American Cancer Society work to fight specific diseases.

However, to the disappointment of many dying people and their relatives, not a single universally known organization has a household-name status while dedicating all its resources to serving the emotional and physical needs of the terminally ill.

The Hemlock Society of the USA strives to assist or to provide information to such individuals, but primarily to those who choose to end their own lives, "assisted suicide."

While I'll delve much more fully into the suicide subject further on, suffice it to say here that people facing a variety of health issues and family problems yearn for definite advice regarding death and dying.

Since the blockbuster 1969 bestseller by Elisabeth Kübler-Ross there have been no additional follow-up, groundbreaking books on this essential topic.

Of course, there have been numerous successful books in recent decades regarding "life after death," a topic that I'll also tackle further on.

Cognizant of the "information void" regarding death during the current era, herein I strive to fill that gap. In doing so I'm bowing to the requests of my many patients who have asked me to pen a timely, incisive book on this vital topic.

James W. Forsythe, M.D., H.M.D.

Even at our birth, death does but stand aside a little. And every day he looks towards us and muses somewhat to himself whether that day or the next will draw nigh.

- Robert Bolt

I cannot possibly stress enough that Kübler-Ross's work remains vital, and her essential research remains the bedrock of my subsequent findings and recommendations chronicled here.

With this understood, I ask readers to please use my own advice that follows as a springboard for addressing their own individual death and dying issues.

While each of us is destined to die someday with virtually no escape, each individual has his or her own unique set of fears, questions, desires and personal issues on the topic.

Mindful of these various unique challenges, let us start out here by realizing that we're all on the same playing field with a predictable outcome—we're all going to die.

The late Leo Buscaglia, the famed bestselling author praised worldwide for his expertise on love, perhaps summarized this best when he once gave advice to a friend.

"Cherish every moment that you have now, because everything will change," Buscaglia said. "If you live long enough, everyone that you know now will be dead by the time you reach your final years. When that happens, all your siblings and cousins, plus your parents, likely will be dead. Although these transitions seem to occur steadily over a period of many years, when looking back during advanced age to you this all will have seemed to have happened in a blink of an eye … Ultimately, like I say, this means that while we're young and middle-aged and seniors, we can appreciate life more if we take time to acknowledge the many blessings in each and every moment."

About Death

We cannot banish dangers but we can banish fears. We must not demean life, by standing in awe of death.

-David Sarnoff

Bolstered by the wisdoms of lifestyle teachers such as Buscaglia, today I'm eager to illustrate the wide, massive and all-encompassing scene that involves death and dying.

Many of my suggestions and observations likely will emerge as highly controversial.

There's a strong chance that many of my philosophies and views on death will be considered all-new, in some instances positions that few if any doctors ever dared broach.

For many, my additional findings might seem basic. Yet I surmise that lots of people likely will end up saying to themselves, "it's all so basic—why didn't I think of that before?"

Understandably, many of us either refuse to or fail to give our own eventual deaths much thought "until the end is near"—that is, if we're "lucky" enough to realize that death is approaching.

The late Timothy Leary, the "tune-in, turn-on, drop-out" guru that I mentioned earlier, served as a prime example of this get-the-info-at-the-last minute behavior.

During the final year before his own death in 1995, while dying from prostate cancer, Leary developed an outline for a book that he planned on the experience, "Design for Dying." The book was released in 1997 two years after Leary's death, which friends filmed at his request for "posterity."

Although Leary's last-minute efforts to teach the world about dying might have been honorable, from my view the effort was "ego-driven, all about him." The man behaved as if his upcoming demise was unique and that the whole world supposedly should take note of what he was experiencing—when in fact death is something we all must face naturally.

James W. Forsythe, M.D., H.M.D.

Tradition demands that we not speak poorly of the dead.
— Daniel Barenboim

Instinctively while I was a teenager for a reason that still remains somewhat mysterious to me today, somehow deep down within my soul I sensed much of my personal and professional future. At the time my heart told me that I would learn about the death process and other vital medical discoveries, eventually teaching the world about my critical findings.

One of my early mentors, an inspiration for me to eventually enter the medical profession, was a doctor—the father of one of my high school classmates in Southern California.

Although living the fast-paced life of a typical youngster, working numerous odd part-time jobs to make ends meet while attending school, as a teenager I still found time to write the manuscript for a book.

"Raising Ruth," was about my experience with my mother. Starting in my early childhood and with increasingly greater responsibilities, I essentially felt as if I was raising my mom—as if I were the mature person in our family, the parent, literally the provider.

The book never was published. Those experiences failed to diminished my deep and full, healthy love for my mom—a highly intelligent and hard-working divorcee.

I played an essential role in caring for my mother until her dying day. Yes, death eventually overcomes us all, even those—obviously—whose children or other close relatives are doctors or medical professionals.

Without health, life is not life; it is only a state of languor and suffering—an image of death.
— Buddha

About Death

So many of my patients have died that—if buried in a single graveyard—their bodies literally would fill some of the largest cemeteries in the United States.

More than merely headstones or decaying objects inside buried boxes, these were the souls of the people I loved professionally and personally.

Truly and to the best of my abilities, I cared for each and every one of them as best as my skills, knowledge and medical criteria would allow at any particular time.

Paradoxically, although fully cognizant of the inescapable fact that death eventually overtakes us all, I wanted each and every one of them to continue living.

Each and every moment without any letup whatsoever, I interacted with every patient on a highly professional level—as all these many thousands of "death and coping experiences" collectively became part of my own manly heart.

People fear death even more than pain. It's strange that they fear death. Life hurts a lot more than death. At the point of death, the pain is over. Yeah, I guess it is a friend.

-Jim Morrison

Every time one of my patients dies, part of me passes away.

When that happens, would my currently surviving patients want me to give up hope for their own potential recovery? Or, would they want me to preserve, to continually find, refine and use effective treatment methods?

Since the obvious answer always remains to push forward in a positive manner, that's precisely what I consciously choose to do—often achieving optimal results.

By now you must realize that although death remains inescapable for us all, human life is a precious gift that must be prolonged as long as possible amid good health.

From my personal and professional view this truism prevails, particularly among individuals who enjoy mobility, fairly keen minds and at least enough vitality to experience life without unnecessary pain.

Fling but a stone, the giant dies.
                                                   -Matthew Green

Instinctively as Mother Nature dictates the vast majority of us want to live as long as possible. To behave otherwise likely would doom our species.

Throughout my career I've only seen a few Stage IV cancer patients give up hope early on the in the process of fighting for their own lives. Each of those instances occurred in the 1970s when only 3 percent of such patients survived while under my care, similar to percentages nationwide.

At the time I remained somewhat perplexed by the decisions of those few individuals to give up their fight far too early. Looking back from today's perspective, however, I realize that perhaps those individuals faced the truth that their survival chances were miniscule.

Setting aside those rare instances, the vast majority of cancer patients faithfully and rigorously follow their physicians' recommendations.

Even in instances where highly poisonous chemo or harmful radiation treatments drastically worsen overall health the vast majority of cancer patients strive to follow doctors' orders—using every ounce of remaining energy that they can muster.

Intellectual growth should commence at birth and cease only at death.
                                                   - Albert Einstein

The overriding goal remains to get as well as possible, for patients with a wide variety of potentially fatal diseases such as

About Death

cancer or critical injuries from accidents.

Thankfully, when such conditions emerge most people possess a basic refusal—denying the probability of death in order to struggle for survival.

Perhaps this is among nature's many ways of motivating doctors to identify, develop or administer likely cures in time to reverse a patient's deteriorating condition.

Indeed, imagine what the health care system would be like if all patients suffering from cancer or other deadly ailments immediately gave up hope or the will to fight.

In essence the extremely rare people who quickly resign themselves to death are at least mentally similar to a baseball player who flat-out refuse to step up to the plate to take his rightful turn at bat. Certainly a player cannot possibly win unless entering the game. The same holds true for patients with cancer or other serious ailments.

The reports of my death have been greatly exaggerated.
- Mark Twain

"I'm alive," often becomes the first thought of patients as they slowly and groggily awaken in hospital recovery rooms following intense surgeries.

People lucky enough to survive horrific train wrecks, plane crashes and auto accidents often immediately get struck by a realization that they escaped death.

Although still emotionally shocked by the sudden trauma such individuals often inquire right away whether other passengers remain alive.

Thankfully, Mother Nature also instills in a vast majority of humans an innate desire and motivation to do whatever possible to help save others.

Particularly in women thanks largely to their inbred desire to care for and nurture others, the desire to assist people in need serves as a primary motivation to become nurses. When first entering their profession, male and female doctors often mention an instinctive desire to help people as among primary reasons for their career choice.

Cowards die many times before their deaths; the valiant never taste of death but once.
- William Shakespeare

As stated earlier, almost every week I get thank-you letters and messages from my patients grateful for my role in "saving" their lives.

Such emotional outpourings often overflow from patients who had not previously expressed intense emotion within my presence or when with my clinic's staff.

Perhaps as humans our basic survival instinct mandates that our minds struggle to help keep the entire body alive for as long as possible.

Without question throughout history people have expressed a renewed appreciation for the own lives following instances where they narrowly escape the grim reaper.

At least from the eyes of many observers, the mark of a true champion emerges when the individual refuses to face the odds against him and ultimately perseveres.

From this view perhaps facing and cheating death becomes somewhat of a sport, at least in a somewhat basic sense. While some lay people or medical professionals might label such an assertion as "hogwash," most are competitive by nature.

Courage is being scared to death...and saddling up anyway.
-John Wayne

Today I would be a billionaire many times over if I had gotten $1,000 for every time someone with advanced Stage IV cancer told me that "doctor, I'm going to fight. I'm going to win against this thing."

In fact, never once in my career of nearly a half century has any patient told me early during the examination process, "I'm going to give up now. There's no use in fighting."

Almost from the get-go, many patients proclaim the fact that they're going to "battle this thing" not only for themselves but for their families and their friends as well.

Much of the time even people without any living relatives or acquaintances take similar attitudes. The yearning to survive invariably dominates feelings of loneliness.

Such attitudes and survival instincts make the job easier for me and for other medical professionals. At least in some instances a positive "winning attitude" becomes essential, even in cases where the doctor has administered the best treatments possible.

As we'll discuss much further later on, a positive, can-do attitude can serve as the integral factor in determining whether an outcome is "life or death."

Death makes angels of us all and gives us wings where we had shoulders smooth as ravens claws.
-Jim Morrison

"Never give up hope," I sometimes tell patients, particularly amid the most harrowing time of their treatment experiences.

As recounted in several of my other books, some patients visiting other doctors, clinics or hospitals are sometimes told to "get your affairs in order."

I tell patients that when and if that ever happens to when visiting another doctor, immediately leave that physician or medical facility and find help elsewhere.

Among the "worst" things that can happen to patients with cancer or other life-threatening conditions is to hear that their doctor has given up all hope for their survival.

James W. Forsythe, M.D., H.M.D.

On some occasions I have "cured" patients after they were told elsewhere that they were *"definitely going to die soon."* Just because your doctor has given up hope on your survival does not mean that you should surrender all such desire to save yourself.

Some of the worst cancers generally considered as "universally fatal" often attack critical organs such as the liver, pancreas, lungs and brain.

Yet I've "cured" numerous such patients. In terms that doctors understand—generally—a patient is considered cured when the cancer goes into remission for a continuous period of at least five years.

The only difference between death and taxes is that death doesn't get worse every time Congress meets.
             -Will Rogers

Far more times than I can remember, I've experienced instances where a patient was "miraculously cured" while virtually on death's doorstep. Under such conditions unless effective treatment is administered the patient would have died within 24 hours.

Faced with such a situation during the final hours before predicted death, some doctors—particularly standard-medicine allopathic physicians—essentially leave the scene rather than attempt to administer desperate "final-hours" treatments. These doctors seemingly disappear while leaving the few remaining chores to nursing staffs.

Sadly, in some of these instances the patient could have rebounded and eventually recovered, resuming healthy, happy and productive life. Lots of the times, I suspect, the doctors who bolted lacked the knowledge, expertise or capability of administering non-toxic natural remedies such as those that homeopaths can provide.

"Never give up hope, until such time as the end comes," I tell some patients. "If you surrender the end will definitely come.

About Death

Always remember that your suffering can end, boosted by a sudden or gradual reversal toward improved health—starting at a time when all hope might otherwise seem lost."

Certainly as a medical professional I'm among those convinced that so-called "fate" can be cheated, refusing to accept the age-old adage that "when your time for death has come, it has arrived and there is no escaping whatsoever."

In spite of everything I believe that people are really good at heart. I simply can't build up my hopes on a foundation consisting of confusion, misery and death.
-Anne Frank

Even amid the continuous need to remain positive, no doctor could or should issue a 100-percent guarantee that you'll experience a "cure" from cancer or any other type of sometimes-fatal disease.

As a seasoned medical professional, I never have or never will make such a promise, particularly to those suffering from worse-phase Stage IV cancer.

"But doctor, aren't you being hypocritical in stating this," some people might proclaim. "How can you possibly insist that cancer patients never give up hope, while at the same time refusing to guarantee their survival?"

Well, despite the greatest, most valiant efforts of a physician, Mother Nature sometimes dictates that a patient's health take a certain fast-track pathway toward a final breath.

Even while undergoing the most diligent, high-tech or natural care imaginable, a patient can sometimes take a sudden, horrible turn for the worse. The many possible outcomes might include everything from sudden death by heart attack to stroke or hemorrhage.

Many types of patients, not just those with cancer, are

impacted by such hazards. Everyone from people suffering heart ailments to people in early-stage Parkinson's Disease face the possibility of sudden death. Remember, undeniably, such an eventual outcome will eventually impact each and every one of us—the ultimate guarantee.

In this world nothing can be said to be certain, except death and taxes.
-Benjamin Franklin

Chapter 7
Death Defined

Although the answer might seem obvious, people living in all stages of life from the young to those in advanced age need to know what death actually "is."

At this juncture a critical need emerges to the dying process on a scientific level.

Without delving into streams of unnecessary jargon that only medical students and doctors need to know, all people need basic knowledge regarding death—whether currently healthy or suffering from serious illness.

With equal importance a need arises to explain "what life is," without which death could never be possible.

As explained by scientists, "life" exists within any object that has a "signaling and self-sustaining biological process" that functions until death.

Life permeates any object that has organisms, tissues, and cells currently in the process of digestion and reproduction—while also interacting with organisms.

__Death comes to all, but great achievements build a monument which shall endure until the sun grows cold.__

- Ralph Waldo Emerson

Similar to the way that many other people feel, to me life encompasses far more than merely biological functions.

For me, life is the smile of my wife Earlene, coupled with her infectious laugh, boundless energy and intelligence as a widely respected leader.

On an even grander scale, life emits rainbows marking its fortitude and gracefulness whenever I see my patients smile, chuckle and crack jokes as they display courage.

Life smiles upon this world whenever my dedicated and highly trained clinic personnel dutifully care for each patient—treating everyone as lovable individuals.

Yes, far more than merely a biological function, in order to be worthwhile life can only exist for humans when they experience emotion—the good and the bad. Mostly I see such innate reactions multiply when witnessing a person's passion for their personal interests, their love of family and their desire for fulfillment.

Do the thing we fear, and death of fear is certain
-Ralph Waldo Emerson

To me, life shows its boundless and endless possibilities when Earlene and I share ice cream with our grandchildren or play games with the youngsters. Enjoying barbecues and going for walks with relatives on the beach at Lake Tahoe energize the heart, mind and soul.

My heart and mind react to the life force that flows into our universe, upon seeing one of my patients cry or on those occasions when I give good news: "You're in remission."

A highly cooperative yet competitive man by nature, I enjoy the lively, frustrated expressions my morning tennis buddies emit on those occasional morning when I happen to beat them.

Surely, these fellows become full of life, cherishing the hurt look on my face when I lose, or perhaps they also enjoy looking at my expressions whenever I win.

With equal intensity I suppose, I recently felt more alive and vibrant than ever when recovering from hip-replacement surgery. As indicated earlier, many of my countless patients have already

About Death

taught me that the physical recovery process becomes possible and accelerates when we remain positive.

It is not death that a man should fear, but he should fear never beginning to live.
-**Marcus Aurelius**

Other than my tight personal or professional bonds with Earlene, our family, staff, patients and many friends, for me life blossoms in all its glorious possibilities whenever I "save" people, whenever I learn, and whenever I teach others.

Indeed, life has absolutely no meaning or impact whatsoever unless we first experience the best or even some of the worst of the unlimited possibilities of our limited time here on earth.

In this vain, I experienced fear that raced through my mind—generating physical reactions that engulfed my entire body—immediately before my arrival in Saigon in early 1969 during the height of the Vietnam War. As I rode with more than 100 other soldiers in a large military aircraft, our plane was fired upon by the enemy.

The unavoidable reality of my potential imminent death at least temporarily robbed me of the ability to think clearly. Luckily for me and for my comrades, our plane landed safely without sustaining damage as all of us escaped injury.

At least in a sense, my emotional reaction at the time was somewhat like what many of my patients have endured over these many years. As humans, we fear the unknown, particularly real or perceived attackers whom we lack any immediate ability to flee from, or have the capability of destroying. Whether by disease, war or recovering from injuries, whenever confronted amid the "heat of battle" we begin to appreciate and acknowledge our own lives with greater fervor than ever before.

James W. Forsythe, M.D., H.M.D.

Each death is a little life: every waking and rising a little birth, every fresh morning a little youth, every going to rest and sleep a little death.
-Arthur Schopenhauer

So, on this particular day are you in fear of losing your own life in the near future?

Whether you're currently facing down potential death or enjoying vibrant health, what does "life" mean to you at this very moment?

Remember, before clearly and fully understanding what "death is," we must first understand, and appreciate or at least acknowledge the pain and joy of our own lives.

As all of us know, life is invariably "hard and challenging," particularly among people who live into our 20s and beyond.

Under the dictates of Mother Nature, life brings conflict and disagreements with other people, along with sudden and unexpected hurdles that often seem insurmountable.

To be sure, as the age-old sayings tell us, "No one ever guaranteed that life would be easy," and capping this off as numerous poets have proclaimed, life itself is a "bucket of tears."

Fully cognizant of these universal challenges facing us all, I would be among the worst kind of fools if I tried to proclaim that death is always easy or that by merely "having a positive attitude, everything will turn out okay."

Let us beware of saying that death is the opposite of life. The living being is only a species of the dead, and a very rare species.
-Friedrich Nietzsche

Mindful of these constant truisms, for you as an individual the need arises to ponder what life means to you.

At this particular moment, whether healthy or suffering from disease or injuries, while learning about death the need arises to "take stock of your personal situation."

Perhaps you're currently frightened after recently being told that you have cancer or another serious disease. Maybe you have just discovered that physicians have diagnosed you as having incurable and ultimately fatal Lou Gehrig's disease, amyotrophic lateral sclerosis—also commonly known as ALS.

Or, perhaps at this very moment you're a prisoner sitting on Death Row, waiting to die on a pre-set date, perhaps still holding onto a smidgen of hope that your lawyer will win a stay of execution.

Whatever your particularly situation, as I've already indicated, you first need to understand your own life in order to "know death," and thereby eventually look your eventual demise straight in the eye.

When your time comes to die, be not like those whose hearts are filled with fear of death, so that when their time comes they weep and pray for a little more time to live their lives over again in a different way. Sing your death song, and die like a hero going home.

-Tecumseh

"That's one book that I'll be sure to avoid," one person, a senior citizen, recently said in a serious tone upon being told that this book was about to be published.

Like this or not, if national statistics bear out the woman likely be facing the end of her life within the next few years. An added challenge emerges when considering the fact that her husband of more than a half century is five years older at age 80

Sadly, I've seen similar scenarios countless times.

Although exceptions occur, at least judging by what I've witnessed, the people who insist on remaining in denial about death suffer the greatest mental anguish amid this unavoidable process.

Conversely, those who face death, who strive to understand and accept its power, often end up feeling a far greater sense of calmness and peace throughout this transition.

For a dying person's living healthy relatives who are destined to outlive them, such a strategy can fortify coping mechanisms—thereby enabling them to endure and to move forward with their own lives in positive direction.

Ordinary people seem not to realize that those who really apply themselves in the right way to philosophy are directly and of their own accord preparing themselves for dying and death.

-**Socrates**

Mindful of the essential need to understand death, you should seize this opportunity—here and now—to ponder what your own life has meant to you.

What are the physical things and the emotional experiences that you have gotten the most pleasure from so far in your own life?

Without becoming overly emotional or spiteful, inspect the reverse side of the same proverbial playing card. What things or experiences have hurt you the most, caused the greatest physical or mental pain, or generated the worst fear deep within your heart?

Even more specifically, when was the last time that you told someone near and dear to you that you truly and wholly love them?

Right now, at this very moment, think of the precise way that your heart felt at the supreme, penultimate moments with the people that you cared about—either romantically or in a platonic sense.

With just as much zest, ponder those specific experiences or instances when you've interacted with others in a hateful manner and in a loving way as well. Think of your many disappointments, your pride at accomplishments—if any—and also about your

About Death

unfulfilled dreams that might have "come true."

Ultimately, when pondering and honestly answering questions such as these, almost everyone wise enough to face these realities generates this similar conclusion: "My life today is what it is—nothing can change what has happened, or what eventually will occur and should occur as Mother Nature dictates. I will die."

We are dying from over-thinking. We are slowly killing ourselves by thinking about everything. Think. Think. Think. You can never trust the human mind anyway. It's a death trap.
-Anthony Hopkins

Upon motivating yourself to face, acknowledge and accept these realities, the ideal time emerges to learn about the process of death.

Through many years of direct experience with such situations, this transition has what I have categorized as having three distinct aspects. The scientific, spiritual and emotional elements come to play to varying degrees in almost every instance.

Many hundreds or thousands of times, far more occasions than I can specifically count, I have gently held the hands of people as they took their final breaths

I have been present when many relatives and friends surrounded and attempted to emotionally comfort their beloved as the person died. The wailing, yelling, muttering and calmness seem to span the vast potential spectrum of human emotions.

Even when death has been anticipated for a long time, among some survivors the "passing away" comes as a shock—electrifying and assaulting the mind, body and spirit.

Particularly as seen by the eyes of an inexperienced or untrained observer, additional reactions might seem perplexing or even somewhat scary.

Rare occasions involve survivors who fail to show any emotional reaction whatsoever, immediately before, during and after witnessing the death of a loved one of many decades. Vacuuming a living room rug or washing the dinner dishes likely would get a far more emotional reaction from such individuals.

Either shock or ignorance, or perhaps a combination of both instills within the hearts of such individuals a motivation to appear as if cold and uncaring.

Death is not the worst that can happen to men.
-**Plato**

An even wider spectrum of reactions and behaviors becomes possible among dying people. Contrary the mistaken belief throughout much of society, at least for a time during their last day of life many terminally ill people are able to move and to speak.

Particularly among those who have either refused to or failed to acknowledge and accept their pending deaths beforehand, some terminal people on their final day toss, turn and flail their limbs about. Screaming or at least some form of grunting occasionally emerges, as these individuals allow fear to grip their dying hearts and to seize control of their psyches.

Some of the most difficult situations to witness in those final hours and moments involve relatives who similarly allow themselves to "lose their minds."

Rather than being there as a strong and loving support for their dying relative or friend, such individuals worsen the situation for the terminally ill or fatally injured.

Imagine being on your own deathbed, wailing and flailing in a pointless attempt to save your own life—all while someone you know behaves in a similar way in regard to your pending demise. This worsens an already harrowing situation.

Madame, all stories, if continued far enough, end in death, and he is no true storyteller who would keep that from you.
- **Ernest Hemingway**

About Death

Phrases such as "Kill me, please," or "I want to die right now; end my pain" sometimes are uttered weakly or screamed full force by the soon-to-be-departed.

Invariably, during the vast majority of situations, however, I'm pleased to report that the initial findings of Elisabeth Kübler-Ross still hold true. Just as she proclaimed, the vast majority of deaths lack such dramatic screaming or movements, but instead entail a rather sedate situation of "passing away."

Judging by the many deaths that I've witnessed, the person passing away exhibits either no signs or at the very least minimal symptoms of suffering physical pain.

Regrettably, however, the vast majority of these people failed or refused to acknowledge the upcoming event beforehand.

The integral process of acknowledging their own lives will end sometimes generates what I call "a more peaceful death."

Life is a process of becoming, a combination of states that we have to go through. Where people fail is that they choose to elect a state and remain in it. This is a kind of death.
-Anis Nin

Chapter 8

Certifying Death

After fully acknowledging your own life's many diverse and intermixed emotions and experiences, the next phase that I recommend is to develop a clear and focused understanding of what happens on a scientific level when death occurs.

Doctors and biologists tell us that they have developed three definitions or determinations of when death happens. Each society, culture or government worldwide chooses which definition of "death" to accept, hinged on its own law and traditions:

Brain death: All activity and particularly electrical impulses stop functioning within the brain, considered by physicians as an irreversible condition.

Vital signs: Some cultures still define death as when breathing and heartbeats stop. Yet the development of cardiopulmonary resuscitation or CPR, plus life support systems and organ transplants has motivated many societies to modify their definition of death.

Largely as a result of the fogginess and confusion regarding the cessation of heart and lung functions, doctors in most cultures have steadily begun to define death as the point after which the brain's electrical activity ceases.

The bodies of some people who have suffered brain death continue to remain "alive" or still possessing viable organ functions, sometimes made possible thanks to life support machines.

When many young or middle-age people reach this stage, following a sudden injury or fatal wound they're considered potential organ donors, often until the moment medical personnel turn off life support machines.

Death is a challenge. It tells us not to waste time...It tells us to tell each other right now that we love each other.
-Leo Buscaglia

Many people, particularly those who failed to pay attention in high school biology class, become amazed to learn that each of us has been continually dying since birth.

Throughout each phase of life all of us from the very young to the extremely old experience the daily deaths of billions of our bodily cells.

This means on a scientific level that the dead cells have stopped functioning as self-sustaining biological objects, no longer using oxygen and no longer reproducing.

The number of our cells that die daily is so massive that our bodies excrete or remove many of these dead cells when we perspire, urinate or have bowel movements.

Many of the remaining dead cells flake off or fall away relatively unnoticed from the surface of our skin. Within many cultures this biological process generates the vast majority of what many people typically call "house dust."

Yes, as bizarre as this might sound, it's true.

When you vacuum or sweep your living room or bedroom, especially tucked-away places like the junctures of walls and floors or those hard-to-reach places behind furniture, much of the dust is actually the "human remains" from your own body, or from your relatives or house guests.

James W. Forsythe, M.D., H.M.D.

At a formal dinner party the person nearest death should always be seated closest to the bathroom.
                                                                        -George Carlin

    The realization that we've been biologically dying since birth can bring mental comfort to people who worry, "What will I feel like after I die? Will I still suffer pain?"

    For those disbelieving in the house-dust explanation, there's an additional method to demonstrate that no pain or sensation occurs in your cells that have died.

    The next time you take a bath spend at least a few minutes soaking before scrubbing any part of your body. Then, use your fingers to rub the spaces between your toes. You can also use the knuckle of your thumb to rub the skin of your heel.

    Particularly if this is done when taking the first bath in at least a few days, miniscule specs of your skin will leisurely float the surface of the bathwater. Many people will experience seeing huge sections of this matter float on the water.

    Now, form your hands into cup-like spheres and let the dead skin rest in your palms. What you're seeing and possibly feeling now with your sensitive fingertips and hand skin is a "dead" former part of you—which lacks any ability to feel pain.

No evil can ever happen to a good man, either in life or after death
                                                                        -Plato

    Without that "dead" part of you that you wash away while bathing or sweep into a dustpan with a broom, you never would have lived.

    Yes, if your health now permits and if you want, you can go out tonight and dance or watch a movie, or enjoy a good meal

About Death

chatting with friends.

All the while perhaps more than ever before, particularly if you have not learned this until now, you now "live" although a part of you has "died."

Taking this realization a step further, you can and should acknowledge the fact that although you live at this moment someday your entire body will die en masse.

So, the need for at least a small bit of repetition here helps drive this point home into the psyche. You are living, although you are dead and you will die in a biological sense. To avoid this reality and to think otherwise is tantamount to cheating yourself and your family as well.

Men are convinced by your arguments, your sincerity and the seriousness of your efforts only by your death.
- Albert Camus

Throughout the ages wise people have called the death of a single individual a "tragedy," while the simultaneous deaths of thousands or millions are a mere "statistic."

Whether admitting this or not, you and I—all of us—will become a statistic someday.

Why?

Well, to put this into clear focus that everyone can understand, an average of 150,000 people die each day, according to the World Health Organization.

This means in a never-ending process nearly two people die somewhere worldwide every single second.

Yes, the hour of your death will arrive today or perhaps tomorrow, or maybe next week, or next month, next year or within decades—but it will come.

When that occurs, your biological cells will become like the house dust that you've swept away or that you've eliminated from your body in the restroom.

The safest course is to do nothing against one's conscience. With this secret, we can enjoy life and have no fear from death.
                                               -Voltaire

Certainly to this point in life you have never bothered to weep daily in grief for the billions of cells that die within your body every day.

Within healthy children, young people and the middle-aged, the continually dying cells are reliably, predictably and efficiently replaced by new but similar organisms.

The probability of overall bodily death among seniors increases, a sharp reversal from their earlier stages of life. As we age cell replacement gradually becomes increasingly inefficient, unreliable and hap-hazard in an unpredictable manner.

This is precisely why, according to the World Health Organization, about two thirds of the 150,000 people who die daily—or about 100,000 of them—die from "old age."

In scientific terms this is "senescence," commonly called old age. The decrease or disruption of the cell-replication processes wrecks and eliminates healthy metabolism. This, in turn, causes the entire body to eventually deteriorate and die.

As a well-spent day brings happy sleep, so a life well-spent brings happy death.
                                               -Leonardo da Vinci

Perhaps even more than most people, as a seasoned physician I've learned first-hand that almost all of us—those enough to acknowledge that their eventual deaths are inescapable—want to die in extreme old age. Preferably this would occur painlessly, well past 100 years old while asleep.

About Death

Yet the Grim Reaper uses the excuse of a wide variety of causes to snatch away each of us. Besides accidents, suicide, murder and natural disasters, the most prevalent causes usually hinge on potentially fatal diseases and adverse physical conditions.

When your "time" eventually arrives, either you'll experience an extremely slow and very painful death, or you'll die suddenly—maybe even unexpectedly.

At least every few months or so, much of the world's population expresses shock and surprise upon learning of the sudden, unexpected death of a big-name celebrity.

But actually, at least in a biological sense this is no big news, since thousands of other people suffer similar unexpected fates daily.

We get into the habit of living before acquiring the habit of thinking. In that race which daily hastens us toward death, the body maintains its irreparable lead.
― Albert Camus

Sociologists and statisticians report that more than 7 billion people now live on earth.

Each and every one of these individuals is in the exact same proverbial boat, at least in the shared experience—a realization that all of us will eventually die.

So, we as individuals and as a society can view this overall spectrum as if a deep-dark tragedy or conversely as a natural and predictable process.

An analysis of the big statistics helps put the overall situation into perspective. The 150,000 people who die daily constitute about one-thousandth of one-percent of the world's total population.

To their credit for the most part, except for intermittent and widespread instances to the contrary, almost every country and culture claims to place great value on human life.

James W. Forsythe, M.D., H.M.D.

It is not the end of the physical body that should worry us. Rather, our concern must be to live while we're alive—to release our inner selves from the spiritual death that comes from living behind a façade designed to conform to external definitions of who and what we are.
~ **Elisabeth Kübler-Ross**

Chapter 9

The Good, the Bad and the Ugly

As you're undoubtedly aware by now, I'm among those who agree wholeheartedly that human life reigns as the most precious gifts that the universe can bestow.

Yet death can and often does emerge as highly valued or "much-welcomed" as well, particularly in instances where the departed suffered extreme pain caused by disease or injury.

Indeed, although I strive professionally, morally and spiritually from preventing such an outcome for any of my patients, the "passing away" of the body eventually occurs.

Whether you refuse to acknowledge or admit this or not, death maintains its well-deserved reputation as the "great equalizer."

Besides robbing us of the very young and the extremely old, death takes away the rich and the poor, the wicked and the kind, the hateful and the loving.

At least some of the time death serves as a blessing by guaranteeing to rid our world of the most hated tyrants in history. The likes of Adolf Hitler and similar devils have moved onward to where they belong, the eternal fire of hell.

A belief in hell and the knowledge that every ambition is doomed to frustration at the hands of a skeleton have never prevented the majority of human beings from behaving as though death were no more than an unfounded rumor.
                                        -Aldous Huxley

Sworn to protect the privacy of my individual patients, while withholding names I'm able to say that some of them have been world-renowned celebrities.

My treatments have "cured" some famous individuals, delaying their eventual demise. Other big-name stars under my care were not so fortunate.

Like those of us who are relatively unknown to the world, some of these celebrities died bravely and courageously, with honor. Others remained gripped with fear, bitter until the end—displaying their vulnerability and humanity.

At least in the overall scheme of things, death plays no favorites—other than the fact that some people can afford medical care, while others lack funds or insurance necessary to receive life-extending treatments.

As I professionally observe people face these issues on a daily basis, I cannot help think of the iconic fictional character Scarlett O'Hara from Margaret Mitchell's classic Civil War novel, "Gone With the Wind," the basis for the blockbuster 1939 movie starring Vivian Leigh and Clark Gable.

Every time this young woman needs to face critical life-and-death, life-changing issues—she vows to essentially "think about it tomorrow." Well, many people today suffering from advanced Stage IV cancer or other potentially mortal conditions take a similar strategy to Scarlett's in death-related matters—ultimately performing a disservice to themselves and to their families. This is often called denial.

About Death

If a man can bridge the gap between life and death, if he can live on after he's dead, then maybe he was a great man.
-James Dean

To gain further insight into the death process, your next assignment entails contemplating your current place within the cosmos.

While pondering this, keep in mind that every man, woman and child who has ever lived on this earth has produced human biological waste. Many of these fertilizers have, in turn, served as nutrients in enabling new life to form.

Like this or not, throughout your entire lifetime you have eaten many thousands of plants, plus the remains of animals if you are not a vegetarian.

All this points to the fact that countless life forms have died in the past, paying the ultimate price so that you can remain alive. Indeed, humans are perhaps the most efficient, most prolific parasites in world history.

A parasite is any living creature, particularly small animals and miniscule cells that thrive biologically by continually living off of other life forms.

Today, as an integral part of this continuous cycle as dictated by rules that nature has set, you never cry about the plants and animals that have perished on your behalf. In all likelihood for the rest of your life you'll never shed a single tear for them.

Ironically, as human beings we cry for ourselves as our own time approaches, thinking as if somehow we should consider ourselves "above it all"—more precious than the countless plants and animals that we have eaten Our coming deaths are "merely" a natural, predictable part of this cycle.

James W. Forsythe, M.D., H.M.D.

There is no lonelier man in death, except the suicide, than the man who has lived many years with a good wife and then outlived her. If two people love each other there can be no happy end to it.

-Ernest Hemingway

Scientists tell us that humans are among only a handful of today's living creatures on earth with the ability of self-awareness. This designation indicates that we know of our existence, just like elephants, certain species of monkeys, dolphins, some whales and a small variety of birds.

Unlike those creatures, people possess the ability to make integral plans for the future and to predict and control a wide variety of possible outcomes.

Certainly, largely due to our continual denial of our future demise, "death" and "die" hail as big, extensive and powerful words. The mere utterance or writing of these terms sends fright or an intense sense of denial into almost every person.

Quite disturbingly from my view, our individual and collective fear has motivated countless people to avoid uttering the word "die" at almost any cost.

Instead, foolish fears have motivated people to use the terms "passing away" or "passing." This strategy of denial is supposedly designed to make people feel better about the situation, as if we're supposed to be convinced that nothing every happened.

Look, I don't want to wax philosophic, but I will say that if you're alive you've got to flap your arms and legs, you've got to jump around a lot, for life is the very opposite of death, and therefore you must at the very least think noisy and colorfully, or you're not alive.

-Mel Brooks

About Death

"Oh, he passed away," people say these days, unlike just a few decades ago when the vast majority of us used the word "died."

Selfish and destructive, our nation's profit-oriented media has compounded this problem, devilishly enabling society to exacerbate our collective denial regarding death.

As a prime example, consider transitions that have impacted the obituary pages of newspapers across the USA, online and in paper printed form.

Until the 21st Century, as dictated by the industry-wide policies of journalists to "stick" to the facts, most obituaries were embossed with the direct, to-the-point, cut-the-bull words like "died," "killed," "murdered," "drowned" or "electrocuted." Even today, standard journalism rules at almost every news organization dictate that reporters and editors use such words in stories involving death.

Yet particularly during the past decade, greedy or profit-driven media companies stopped publishing obituaries free of charge about average people.

As a replacement, newspapers began assessing fees for surviving families to pay for the publishing of obituaries about their loved ones.

Death is not the greatest loss in life. The greatest loss is what dies inside us while we live.
-Norman Cousins

Locked in denial, due to the newspaper's collective greed in charging for pre-written obituaries, families got saddled with the chore of writing and paying for the publication of obituaries.

As a result, the chances of seeing words like "died" or "murdered" are seemingly about 1 million-to-one in today's standard newspaper print or online death notices. Instead, we see phrases such as "passed away," "passed," "crossed over," "was greeted" or "taken into the hands of the Lord."

From my view as a health care professional who deals with

death on a daily basis, such terminology is harmful and destructive for all of society.

Many people might choose to get angry toward me for proclaiming this, but survivors and their families need to clearly face what will happen or what has occurred.

On a broader scale, propagating such propaganda about "passing" only serves to exacerbate society's unnecessary fears, confusion and denial about death.

To do otherwise, to use phrases indicating that the departed loved one "simply walked out a door" performs a disservice for us all.

Instead, we should take a straight-forward approach rather than skirting around the subject by saying matter-of-factly that the person "left us," taking a direct approach would be best of all.

Life is pleasant. Death is peaceful. It's the transition that's troublesome.
                                                                -Isaac Asimov

Grief emerges as a natural and expected reaction among survivors.

Using fluffy terminology at all times might prevent families and friends from facing up to the fact that the deceased person "didn't just leave us, he's gone for good."

To do otherwise is to invite potential psychological disaster among surviving close relatives, surviving spouses or entire families.

As a prime example, consider what happened to a middle-aged friend of mine, Duane, and his numerous siblings.

When Duane was five years old his infant brother died in a tragic household accident just short of his first birthday. Under the suggestion and encouragement of Duane's parents, a doctor administered powerful sedatives to him and his siblings.

Duane and his catatonic brothers were so drugged up that they didn't regain any sense of mental reality until the huge wake three days after the accident. Confused and disoriented upon entering the party, my friend and his living brothers were told at the time that their dead sibling had "passed away" and crossed over to the other side.

From that point forward, no one ever discussed what had happened. Wayne and his siblings were never taught to say the words "death" or "die," but were instead taught to engulf themselves in a deep, relentless and seemingly inescapable world of denial.

It wasn't until a few decades later that subsequent tragedies struck the family. Duane's siblings suffered mental challenges or fell into drug addictions, which they later admitted were actually warped attempts to cope with or understand their little sibling's death from long ago.

Death is a relief from the impressions of the senses, and from desires that make us their puppets, and from the vagaries of the mind, and from the hard service of the flesh.

~ **Marcus Aurelius**

As a doctor I've seen countless instances where a family's insistence on denying death has eventually led to extreme personal and mental issues.

Rather than cry or scream in anger, potentially healthy emotional reactions, some survivors choose to obliterate their minds with drugs, delve full force into alcoholism, or write fluffy obituaries riddled with phrases like "passed away" or "crossed over."

Some survivors might argue that for them these actions are a healthy, understandable and predictable method of doing their best to cope.

Amazingly, a number of people also seem to insist that continued denial is a good and effective strategy, the best tactic imaginable.

To them I say, "Face the truth and you will turn out better

in the long run. Living in denial or delving in substance abuse prevents you from experiencing life to the fullest—while also robbing yourself of the ability to learn from the situation."

We all pay for life with death, so everything in between should be free.
                                                           -Bill Hicks

As a doctor I'm a "realist," fine-tuned to deal with the facts head-on every day. Largely as a result, I refrain from going into my own denial regarding society's intense fear of facing almost any issue regarding death.

Simply telling you here that we should refrain from erecting barriers that allow us to deny death can never change what is occurring today.

Bowing toward their one-true god, Ignorance, and choosing to make "fear" their lifelong master, people will continue using "passed away" phrase in obituaries.

Sadly, on a much broader scale, such terms have permeated throughout much of society, at such a voluminous level that nothing can stem the tide.

Religious leaders that we're supposed to look up to and admire have increasingly started using these fluffy terms during eulogies. This, in turn, essentially gives church-goers an unspoken go-ahead, a signal that it's OK to delve into a world of denial.

Further compounding the issue, I've noticed a steadily increasing number of obituaries in recent days proclaiming that a "closed casket funeral" is planned. Readers seeing this are supposed to embrace the indirect, clandestine message that "everything will be okay if I attend—I won't have to see a body, and I can remain in denial."

When we have lost everything, including hope, life becomes a disgrace, and death a duty.
                                                           -W.C. Fields

About Death

The hosts of popular TV talk shows and radio programs have either unwittingly or unknowingly chosen to worsen the problem.

Chats with popular or world-famous guests that delve into deceased loved ones or friends are now marked with breezy phrases such as "he has left us," or when the "person crossed over." Even psychics on popular reality TV shows refrain from uttering "die," "dead" or "death."

Steadily, any attempt to directly and openly discuss death throughout our society has become a definite, almost unforgivable sin.

On the flip side of this proverbial coin, speaking in terms of denial has gradually become the politically correct language in almost all instances.

Anyone who would dare speak the truth about death, to openly acknowledge such terms, would be deemed as wicked, heartless and perhaps even evil.

In the process, the bulk of society seems to proclaim, "How dare you or anyone force me to face and acknowledge this issue. The way you're talking, in such blunt and direct terms is nothing short of offensive. Shame on you, for saying 'die.'"

Because I could not stop for death, He kindly stopped for me; the carriage held but just ourselves and immortality.
                                                               -Emily Dickinson

This endless depressing trend leaves me somewhat mystified and perplexed, although I remain a pragmatist and a realist.

The situation becomes increasingly mystifying when considering the fact that we live in a society where technology affords instant global communication to almost everyone.

People always used words like "die" and "dead" just a few decades ago before the advent of social Web pages, cell phones, texting, emails and online videos.

Paradoxically, along with the spread of these technologies

society has steadily and gradually chosen to push its head deep into the proverbial sand.

Rather than use these electronic devices for the betterment of everyone in death-related matters, at least outwardly we're collectively diving deeper into our own sense of denial.

No matter how prepared you think you are for the death of a loved one, it still comes as a shock, and it still hurts very deeply.

-**Billy Graham**

Chapter 10
Modern Communication Worsens Issues

Based on the many real-life cases I've witnessed, people during the final phase of the 1900s coped better with their pending deaths or with the deaths of loved ones, as compared to the vast majority of such instances in the 21st Century.

The vast majority of people more than 13 years ago dealt much more directly with death than people do today.

At least judging by what I've witnessed, most people through the 1990s did a far better job at coping with death and moving forward in a positive direction.

By contrast, most of today's grievers—particularly the young and those in the early middle-age years, mentally lock up, freeze and go into denial when death gets mentioned.

Perhaps prior to the advent of cell phones, text messaging, Facebook and Twitter most people gained valuable real-life experience by directly interacting with each other.

By contrast, for many individuals coping with death today, the most intimate interaction they experience on a regular basis involves clicking a computer mouse or pushing cell phone text buttons.

Shrinking away from death is something unhealthy and abnormal which robs the second half of life of its purpose.
-Carl Jung

James W. Forsythe, M.D., H.M.D.

Through the early 1990s, people needing to convey "bad news" about previous or pending deaths were forced to telephone each other, track each other down in person, ask intermediaries to convey messages, compose handwritten letters or send telegrams.

These personal interactions forced people to share tears, argue in person if necessary about funeral arrangements or buckling under to personally call a long-lost relative that they always despised or wanted to avoid.

Like this or not, these limitations in communication forced people to be with one another or at least to talk directly. Although there were numerous exceptions, overall this process forced people to hone their mental-coping skills.

Today's gadgets obliterated much of our ability to satisfy a basic human yearning that most people possess—the process of being with and sharing with other people, particularly during rough times.

Today we notice death postings on Facebook or elsewhere online, instead of being able to grieve openly and fully, or to share our own fears or concerns while dying.

Watching a peaceful death of a human being reminds us of a falling star; one of a million lights in a vast sky that flares up for a brief moment only to disappear into the endless night forever.

-Elisabeth Kübler-Ross

The Internet has numbed the minds of many, particularly those dealing with death. Some people are guilty of typing seemingly meaningless, empty words of condolence.

Proclaiming that "I've done my part," lots of us refrain from attending memorial services. Instead, the choice involves quickly posting a few words on funeral home Websites.

Those who argue that such a reaction should be considered perfectly understandable in today's hectic world need to remember that "people need each other."

About Death

We'll have a much more compelling and in-depth discussion on funerals and the grieving process later. For now, suffice it to say that I've witnessed many times when grieving. People who find the courage to cry with loved ones regarding their own approaching deaths, and who grieve together in person usually tend to recover more quickly and fully from that phase of the experience.

Death is the wish of some, the relief of many and the end of all.

-Lucius Annaeus Seneca

Dying people who cry while in my arms or when hugged by relatives often soon start feeling at least somewhat emotionally better—paving the way to cope and to accept.

When a dying person and I touch hands, a universal acceptance of "what is" seems to permeate our universe. Even those who have just cried often emit genuine smiles.

Physically healthy relatives of the dying react the same way when opening up their hearts enough to bond with relatives and acquaintances, or even medical personnel at permissible and acceptable levels.

To do otherwise, ignoring these individuals' emotional needs would be to turn our backs on our own humanity. Whatever spiritual or religious beliefs each of us has, despite any differences we share an undeniable and irreplaceable bond. We need each other.

So, if you're in denial about a dying relative—while relying solely on technology—, then shut off your cell phone and leave the Internet. Instead, go to your loved one now, remembering that someday you likely will need someone to visit you on your deathbed.

Visiting dying people that you love or care about should impress you as essential. After all, where will you want your relatives and friends to be when you're dying—glued elsewhere to their cell phones and the Internet, or with you in person?

Every parting gives a foretaste of death, every reunion a hint of resurrection.
                                                            -Arthur Schopenhauer

Chapter 11
Question: What happens when we die?

While acknowledging your eventual death and appreciating the need to communicate directly in person with others, the next step is to know what happens when we die.

To put this bluntly your body will start to decompose shortly after death, your flesh including vital organs and muscles literally "food for the worms."

The standard practice in the USA and throughout many societies in recent years has been to embalm or cremate the body soon after death—partly to delay or to avoid decomposition.

This might alleviate at least some of your current concerns. Yet depending on your personal circumstances, there could remain a chance you'll die at home alone.

If you die while home alone, your body will begin to literally rot quicker than an apple fallen from a tree, particularly if your body remains untouched for at least a day. The decaying process actually starts immediately upon death, but starts to accelerate about five hours after the final breath.

There's something about death that is comforting. The thought that you could die tomorrow frees you to appreciate your life now.

-Angelina Jolie

Anyone squeamish about this undeniable process can embrace the eternal knowledge that birth and death are integral parts of the circle of life.

As various philosophers, scientists and religions have proclaimed throughout the ages, our bodies started as "nothing" or ash before our birth—and we return to that state.

Billions of humans have already undergone this transition, and countless billions more will follow you on this predictable and reliable pathway.

So, as I've indicated earlier, why should you feel worried or scared when doing so can do absolutely nothing to prevent this eventual outcome?

During the time that it takes you to finish reading this page many people will die. Some were terrified, and others showed courage or even indifference. Most die in obscurity.

Death, so called, is a thing which makes men weep. And yet a third of life is passed in sleep.

- **Lord Byron**

Countless billions of animals also are being slaughtered or dying naturally.

Remember, unless their dead bodies are eaten, burned or injected with preserving chemicals, all deceased mammals decay—a process some people call "rotting," or decomposing.

If you die while under medical care or in a hospital, soon after doctors declare you dead medical professionals will clean your body.

But first any loved ones or friends who request to do so might be given a chance to spend some alone time with your body. Based on what I've witnessed, when that happens some relatives might proclaim that they hated you, that they dearly loved you, or that they never truly knew or understood your true heart at all.

About Death

This is when some mourners cry, appear emotionless or make no attempt to censor their utter happiness that the departed person's physical and mental suffering has ended.

There are, as is known, insects that die in the moment of fertilization. So it is with all joy; life's highest most splendid moment of enjoyment is accompanied by death.
				-Soren Kierkegaard

A much different process engulfs the corpses of people who die alone.

No two human bodies decompose at the same precise rate and manner.

Particularly if you die alone, the rate and specific type of your body's decomposition will hinge on a huge variety of factors. A huge variety of conditions will be involved, including your body weight, frame size and a wide variety of other factors.

Another factor hinges on how long your body remains undiscovered.

Decomposition immediately begins at the precise moment that the heart and lungs stop. This process halts only if those organs "miraculously" resume functioning on their own within several minutes, or following instances where living people successfully resuscitate the individual.

Nothing can be more beautiful than death.
				-Walt Whitman

If your body remains undisturbed for an extended period of many hours, days, weeks or months, it will follow a universal and predictable decomposition process.

When not eaten after death by large predators like coyotes, wolves, wild dogs, hyenas, lions, tigers or bears, the dead bodies of all mammals initially start to decompose in one or both of two ways.

Biotic decomposition occurs due to a natural degradation or destruction of the physical processes or chemical bonds that prevailed during life.

Rather than merely a natural breakdown of substances, the second form of natural decomposition involves an "abiotic" process. Small or microscopic living organisms essentially eat away at or digest the former living matter that once was your living body.

At this very moment while you're alive, countless billions of microscopic creatures are on the surface and even inside of your body. Many cell-sized organisms are living in such places as the liquid in your eyeballs or the internal lining of your entire intestines.

As long as you're alive these miniscule living organisms usually remain harmless or even helpful to your overall health. But as soon as you die a percentage of these living creatures will start assisting in the natural breakdown of your bodily structure.

Even very young children need to be informed about dying. Explain the concept of death very carefully to your child. This will make threatening him with it much more effective.

                                                                                       -P.J. O'Rourke

"Doctor, why do you choose to mention this here?" you might ask.

Well, on the scientific level before delving into spiritual or religious aspects, such a vital revelation becomes necessary in order to mentally cope with our pending deaths before they occur.

Just like when Sergeant Joe Friday often proclaimed in the 1960s TV series, "Just the facts, ma'am," you need to acknowledge these indisputable and unchangeable details.

Any effort to approach the subject otherwise, ensconcing

ourselves in denial, would result in a disservice to us, and to our families. By proclaiming that "there's no monster—the Grim Reaper—on the other side of a door" when such a creature actually is there will never do anything whatsoever to prevent death's eventual appearance.

On the positive side, from the many instances that I've seen, by acknowledging and understanding that proverbial monster now before our deaths, we can actually transform that intruder into a harmless, friendly mouse or even a mere, unnoticeable insect.

I don't fear death because I don't fear anything that I don't understand. When I start to think about it, I order a massage and it goes away.

-Hedy Lamarr

Upon death the "autolysis" process—commonly labeled as "self-digestion"— enzymes already within the body destroy cells at or near where they had been at death.

Contrary to a common misguided myth, the dead cells are not actually digesting themselves. Chemical action fostered by enzymes does this.

As one of the many miracles within nature, autolytic cell destruction sometimes occurs on a limited basis within living people. Only when necessary this helps the living person remove dead or dying cells, clearing a pathway for potential recovery.

The autolysis uses both enzymes and chemicals to break down bodily tissues.

Adding powerful assistance to the overall process, bacteria—much or all of which had already been within the body while the person lived—will generate "putrefaction," which causes the corpse to stink.

James W. Forsythe, M.D., H.M.D.

If we have not been pleased with life, we should not be displeased with death, since it comes from the hand of the same master.

-Michelangelo

The unmistakable, repulsive and unforgettable stink caused by putrefaction often leads people to proclaim: "I smelled something dead nearby."

Particularly in intensely hot, human summertime conditions, atmospheric conditions in subtropical and tropical areas like Southern Florida cause dead bodies to emit a putrefaction odor. The stench sometimes becomes so overwhelming that approaching the corpses becomes extremely difficult or even impossible.

On occasion in those regions senior citizens die naturally when alone in their houses or apartments. Within a few days after the corpses have remained undiscovered, nearby residences must be temporarily evacuated due to temporary, overwhelming smell.

Lots of the time fire departments and police officers arrive, each crew member wearing gas masks while investigating the scene and removing the body. On occasion although death occurred naturally the corpses appear as if melted, large, steamy, greasy mounds of slimy, steamy, oozing green puss.

If I die prematurely I shall be saved from being bored to death by my own success.

-Samuel Butler

Remember, those dead bodies are not by any stretch of the imagination who these people actually were, the soul of them—the life force and the spirit that once signaled to the world that they were alive.

When your death occurs, the body that you leave behind also will lack any visible signals that you once smiled, laughed or cried.

Keep in mind that the decomposition and putrefaction

processes are merely the predictable, scientific outcome within our physical world.

At this juncture while continuing to learn more about the overall death process, please continue to recall our continually dying cells that I mentioned earlier.

From the perspective of the "soul" of you, the "spirit" of you, the body's death is just like those many cells that I already described—the flakes that rose to the surface of the waters from the spaces between your toes while taking a bath.

Upon learning these many specifics of the decomposition process, such knowledge can help you cope at least somewhat with what will invariably transpire.

Death is the king of this world: 'Tis his park where he breeds life to feed him. Cries of pain are music to his banquet.
                                                                        -George Eliot

Immediately before or even during the stinky putrefaction process, fungi and bacteria join in the work of breaking down a corpse—often assisted by scavengers like buzzards, crows and vultures.

Many insects, including blow-flies and flesh-flies, feast on the bodies. Well before this phase, a newly deceased body starts the first of several decomposition stages.

Right after you die, your corpse will be considered "fresh," well before the stink and extensive breakdown of bodily organisms.

Particularly if left unattended within a few hours after you die the corpse will display a discoloration that scientists, morticians and coroners call "livor mortis." Gravity forces bodily fluids that had once been pumped by the circulatory system to accumulate in certain areas of the body—resulting in a change in color.

I know not what others may choose, as for me, give me liberty or give me death.
                                                                        -Patrick Henry

James W. Forsythe, M.D., H.M.D.

On an average of three to six hours after you die unattended, the "livor mortis" phase will begin where muscles stiffen. Medical crews, firefighters or police who initially find your corpse at this stage will have extreme difficulty moving your joints and limbs.

Due to differences in lactic acids at various places throughout the body, the first areas of your corpse to become stiff will be the jaw, eyelids and neck, gradually followed by the various other joints and limbs.

Assuming you remain unfound, about 12 hours after death the level of your corpse's stiffness will peak. From that point the stiffness gradually subsides. Starting around 48 to 60 hours after death the joints and limbs become much easier to move.

Police detectives who find your body likely will use the corpse's level of livor mortis at the time of being discovered to help determined when you died.

The stage of livor mortis also will be used along with other evidence such as witness statements regarding when they last saw you alive.

It is difficult to accept death in this society because it is unfamiliar. In spite of the fact that it happens all the time, we never see it.

-Elisabeth Kübler-Ross

At this juncture, some readers might ask why I choose to occasionally refer to corpses as "you."

Well, at least for many people, acknowledging what can happen helps them to maturely allow the mind to accept the body's current and future places within the ever-changing universe.

Such an educational strategy might ease fears at least somewhat when learning that even when the body is still fresh, autolysis sometimes forms blisters on the skin.

Also during the "fresh" decomposition stage, small cellular aerobic organisms that had already been inside the body quickly

About Death

start relieving the corpse of any remaining oxygen.

This, in turn, clears the way for another type of living miniscule creature, anaerobic cells that do not require oxygen to survive. These invariably originate from deep within the body, primarily the respiratory system and the gastrointestinal tract.

On the plus side, death is one of the few things that can easily be done lying down.
-
                                                                Woody Allen

Anaerobic cells within dead people start creating gases such as ammonia, methane and hydrogen sulfide, which result from the transformation of proteins, lipids and carbohydrates. Organic acids including lactic acid and propanoic acid also are produced.

The inclusion of these substances clears the way for the famous putrefaction stink process. All this actually happens while the body still remains in the fresh stage.

This inter-laps and is followed by the bloating phase, during which the various gasses distend the abdomen while making the cadaver appear bloated.

Adding to the corpse's horrific appearance, the gasses invariably force fluids to move or pulsate out of all available orifices including the nostrils, mouth, anus, ears and pubic area. Sometimes the gas buildup becomes so intense that the body ruptures.

Meantime various colored pigments along with sulfhemoglobinemia are formed when hemoglobin anaerobic bacteria are formed within the intestines. An overall marbled appearance then covers the corpse, the result of various gasses transporting sulfhemoglobin throughout the body.

Death is not the end. There remains the litigation over the estate.
                                                                -Ambrose Bierce

James W. Forsythe, M.D., H.M.D.

At the height of bloating, tissues and natural liquids become frothy; this occurs as a result of the buildup in gasses throughout the body cavity.

At this juncture, assuming your body still remains unfound, the corpse will become a feasting ground for maggots.

These pesky creatures will amass to feast on bodily tissue, wherever they can dine under the skin and thereby causing the hair to detach and fall. This around-the-clock picnic also results in maggots congregating religiously at the natural orifices.

Almost as if wedding party-goers milling about to and fro shortly after the nuptials, the maggots will essentially move casually indoors and outdoors at will—making your body their own proverbial house of worship.

Skin ruptures occur, partly due to this overcrowding coupled with various chemical processes. This enables oxygen to re-enter the body.

These openings enable the maggots to literally take over your entire body as if greedy, heartless and mindless soldiers at the height of a great war. For the body, the nuclear bomb comes in the form of the oxygen that has re-entered the corpse. A new breeding ground for the larvae of maggots and other insects steadily accelerates the body's decomposition as new swarms of warriors dine on the human tissue.

If I think about death more than some other people, it is probably because I love life more than they do.
-Angelina Jolie

The various insects coupled with ongoing chemical reactions within the cells vastly accelerate the decomposition process well past the "fresh" and "bloating" stages.

Now, the "active decay" stage suddenly takes over. Huge sections of the former body disappear, either eaten by insects or deteriorating due to chemical reactions.

About Death

The corpse's various fluids evaporate or get expelled into the surrounding environment. The stink continues as the fluid buildup in the surrounding area generates what biologists and coroners call a "cadaver decomposition island" or CDI.

So much of the body's former flesh has disappeared that the maggots begin to migrate away, leaving pupate or immature offspring.

Within a relatively short period, usually days or several weeks, the active decay phase is replaced by the advanced decay stage. Here, the rapid decay has markedly decreased, lacking any substantial bodily material. Vegetation dies immediately under or near any human body that has reached this stage, due to the various acids and natural chemicals resulting from the decomposition process.

It seems to me that if you or I must choose between two courses of thought or action, we should remember our dying and try so to live that our death brings no pleasure on the world.
-John Steinbeck

Amid the advanced stage of composition, nitrogen increases markedly in the surrounding soil. This is accompanied by changes in pH, along with increases in calcium, magnesium, and potassium and phosphorous.

The "advanced decay" stage is followed by a phase that scientists call "dry remains." The immediately surrounding area sometimes displays a resurgence in vegetation—at or near the cadaver decomposition island.

Only bones, dry skin and cartilage remain from the original cadaver. When exposed to the elements any remains become dry and bleached.

The remains have become mere skeletons at the point where the remaining cartilage and skin disappear or are torn away by wind or curious scavengers.

James W. Forsythe, M.D., H.M.D.

Basing their conclusions on thousands of intense studies, scientists tell us that the decomposition rate is far slower for corpses that have been buried without being embalmed—but only about eight times slower than normal.

It is impossible to experience one's death objectively and still carry a tune.
               -Woody Allen

Chapter 12

The Five Stages of Grief

At this point, upon being struck by the realization that you definitely will die someday and what happens to dead bodies, in all likelihood you'll be positioned to cope better with what Kübler-Ross described as the first of five stages of grief involving death.

As vividly described in her blockbuster 1969 book "On Death and Dying," virtually everyone experiences denial sensations upon contemplating his or her own deaths—and especially when learning from a physician that "your time on earth is extremely limited."

The same reactions hold true among relatives of mortally ill or critically injured people. Many thousands of times I've seen similar reactions among patients and their relatives, particularly in non-cancerous deaths involving other diseases or fatal injuries.

The late Anna Freud, a psychoanalyst and daughter of the famed Sigmund Freud, theorized that the process of denial among humans signals immaturity.

If true, this would indicate—at least from my view—that many of those denying their own upcoming deaths are reverting to a childlike or adolescent mental state.

I would rather die a meaningful death than live a meaningless life.
-Corazon Aquino

From the viewpoint of many people, a person becomes mature

James W. Forsythe, M.D., H.M.D.

upon accepting and acknowledging the many indisputable and universal facts involving life, and ultimately death as well.

By contrast small children and adolescents through the teenage years often refuse to know, acknowledge or accept potentially disturbing details.

Youngsters who hate or refuse to do chores sometimes "win out" in the long run by avoiding those family duties, only to receive rewards such as treats from their "weak or spoiling" parents.

Much more forcefully, toddlers are some of the world's most conniving and successful negotiators. They'll often cry or throw temper tantrums until they get their way, when parents or caregivers eventually grow weary and buckle into demands.

In a sense, at least in many cases, adults who learn of their incurable diseases use denial as a protective measure in a childish way—rather than accepting the truth in a wise, thoughtful and mature manner.

Death is someone you see very clearly with eyes in the center of your heart; eyes that see not by reacting to light, but by reacting to a kind of chill from within the marrow of your own life.
-Thomas Merton

My assertions here should by no means be construed as an attempt to harshly criticize or complain about dying adults who insist on employing irrational denial.

Mother Nature dictates that fear will emerge as a natural reaction, motivating each of us to do whatever possible to survive in most instances—whatever our age.

Perhaps more than merely as an immature reaction as Anna Freud theorized, perhaps denial is a mere protective mechanism employed to help ourselves and others survive.

Amid intense combat many soldiers deny or strive to ignore the fact that they're soon likely to die instantly or become mortally

About Death

wounded. During their intense training prior to engaging in battle many future warriors are trained that "you're already dead."

This training and in-the-field mental strategy essentially hones soldiers into efficient walking and talking combat machines. When under intense enemy fire, some warriors deny or ignore what likely will happen to them—risking their lives to rescue their comrades. Some rescuers pay the "ultimate price," while thinking only of others.

One is still what one is going to cease to be and already what one is going to become. One lives one's death, one dies one's life.
-Jean-Paul Sartre

On the flip side of the same proverbial coin, as I witnessed many times during the Vietnam War some soldiers learn a different sense of denial. This involves mentally dehumanizing the enemy, perceiving adversaries as entities other than human beings.

Such measures might emerge as another coping mechanism, whether dropping a nuclear bomb on tens of thousands of souls in Japan or serving as a prison guard while assisting directly in the execution of a condemned inmate.

Faced to ponder such situations, most people would wonder whether mankind is intrinsically "evil," naturally "good," or somewhere in between—particularly in instances where entire societies dehumanize or minimize the importance of perceived enemies.

As for me, I have witnessed many instances that fully convince my logical mind and my caring heart that overall for the most part people worldwide are "good."

Sociologists have many diverse and often-conflicting theories on this. Some suggest that perhaps many worriers or nations deny that they're killing or oppressing others, a mental and socially acceptable survival mechanism amid entire cultures.

James W. Forsythe, M.D., H.M.D.

Since change is constant, you wonder if people crave death because it's the only way they can get anything really finished.
                                                                -Chuck Palahniuk

Many people suffering from alcoholism, gambling addictions or various other behavioral issues undergo 12-step recovery programs. Mirroring each other, virtually all these systems involve an initial Stage 1 phase where participants acknowledge the issue.

Alcoholics, gamblers, narcotics abusers and sex addicts can only start on their own personal pathways toward mental and physical recovery by first admitting the problem.

The various 12-step programs, organized on a popular and widely known basis, help people suffering from a wide range of other issues such as workaholics, people who hoard and clutter needless things, and those engulfed in co-dependency.

Well, from what I've seen a similar first-phase strategy can go a long way toward generating a wiser and more accepting attitude among the dying and their relatives.

Besides acknowledging their addictions or problems in Step 1, that phase also entails accepting the fact that we are made powerless by an issue such as death—which ultimately has made our lives seem as if unmanageable.

Old age is a tyrant, who forbids, under pain of death, the pleasures of youth.
                                                        -Francois de La Rochefoucauld

Informally called "The Big Book," the 12-step program for recovery was first described in a 1939 book by Bill Wilson and Doctor Bob Smith: "Alcoholics Anonymous: The Story of How More than One Hundred Men Have Recovered from Alcoholism."

Subsequently re-written or re-formed in order to address a variety of addiction and behavioral issues, the 12-step concept very likely could emerge as a formidable tool for dying people, their families and friends.

Based on my research, I've found little or no widespread or regional 12-step programs dedicated to the death and dying process.

Some people might argue in a joking manner that this is a "dying issue for the terminally ill and mortally injured. Most of them will die by the time they even begin to understand the process."

To anyone who would utter such a statement, I would respond to them in a loving, kind and warm way that the mental pain and anguish facing terminally ill people remains just as critical as most other issues that 12-programs are designed to help.

As a society, as relatives and as dying people we also need to remain fully cognizant that modern medical advancement has vastly extended life expectancies among the terminally ill. Just a few decades ago people died much faster on average than they do now, between the time of their terminal diagnosis and their eventual deaths.

Land and sea, weakness and decline are great separators, but death is the great divorcer for ever.
                                                          -John Keats

In her analysis of the initial first phase of the five stages of grief, Kübler-Ross concluded that while in denial most terminally ill people rapidly gain an awareness of the physical objects that they have accumulated.

Described in various online publications and books as a "heightened awareness of possessions," this mental processing tabulates and chronicles everything that will be left behind on this earth after death.

Cognizant of the fact that as a doctor I focus on enabling people to remain alive, most patients and their families never become motivated for me to discuss the denial phase or the four other grieving stages.

Thus, I rarely see or hear directly about these issue, primarily because the bulk of my conversations with them involve the best possible potential outcomes. Remember, as stated earlier, I never tell patients to get their affairs in order.

Nonetheless, I occasionally discuss such issues with patients or their families when requested. Sometimes they bring up these issues immediately after I sincerely ask "How are you doing?" or "Do you have any more questions that I might answer?"

There is nothing which at once affects a man so much and so little as his own death.
-Samuel Butler

The vast majority of patients never bring up the topic of death with me, probably because our focus remains partly on retaining life.

By the time this happens—if at all—most patients who choose to discuss death are those who have progressed into what Kübler-Ross labeled as the second of the five stages of grief. During this phase anger often erupts.

"Why is this happening to me!" such patients often seem to yell, both internally within their own psyches and verbally. As I've seen or heard many times, verifying the conclusions of Elisabeth Kübler-Ross, numerous dying patients lash out at me or at themselves, their families, friends and various medical professionals.

Usually the anger stems from confusion, an inner conflict that generates twisted logic motivating the person to identify or find someone to blame.

Much of the time the anger erupts with the ferocity of a spouting volcano, beginning at the point where the first stage of denial begins to fade. Faced with the reality of what soon will happen, the person begins experiencing raw, uncensored emotions.

About Death

Whether you like it or not, you're forced to come to the realization that death is out there. But I don't fear death, I'm a fatalist. I believe when it's your time, that's it. It's the hand you're dealt.

-Clint Eastwood

Other than yelling, cursing or whining to relatives, dying people within the second stage of the grieving process sometimes choose to scream at me.

Sometimes when this happens the person confronts me verbally within closed-door offices of my clinic. They'll holler and cry in angry tirades, blaming me for supposedly failing to fulfill a promise that never was actually made—to save their life.

This occasionally occurs when symptoms worsen and reach a critical stage after using treatments that have cured a high number of other patients.

Remember, to this day there remains no universal cure for all forms of cancer, although the remission rates experienced by my patients suffering Stage IV of the disease is much higher than the national average.

The intense anger coupled with envious feelings or rage that some dying patients experience amid stage two of the grieving process often hampers attempts to treat them and to care for them.

Pale death, with impartial step, knocks at the hut of the poor and the towers of kings.

-Horace

Numerous dying people become angry at almost anyone who comes into close contact with them, everyone from medical staff personnel to food servers.

Some of these ill people have been known to throw uneaten plates of food across rooms, or intentionally drop their filled bedpans on the floor.

When such instances happen, seasoned medical workers refrain from passing judgment while also remaining emotionally detached from this childish behavior.

For me as an individual doctor, these patients are real, live, wondrous and lovable human beings who still deserve loving care and attention. Much of the time a patient's anger could hamper or prevent treatments that might still have a chance of putting the disease into remission, or perhaps prolonging life.

On rare occasions, relatives of dying people also become angry upon moving past denial, eventually struck by the realization that their loved one soon will leave forever.

Death would not be called bad, O people, if one knew how to truly die.
-Guru Nanak

Similar to the way that the first phase of the 12-step recovery process helps alcoholics and other addicts, the second stage of that strategy also can be used in assisting dying people and their relatives who have become angry.

Remember, as stated earlier, the first phase of 12-step recovery emerges as an obvious tactic in addressing denial. The person acknowledges the situation is "unmanageable."

In the second level of the 12 steps, people recovering from additions or other problems decide to open their hearts and souls up to a higher power. Doing so also can help work wonders for dying people and their grieving relatives.

By opening up to a higher power greater than themselves, the individual acknowledges and opens themselves up to his or her concept of "the creator" or God. Later on we explain the roles that various religions and spiritual beliefs have in dealing with the death and dying process throughout numerous cultures.

For now, in using the second rung of the 12-step strategy, keep in mind that each individual decides what this "higher power" means to him or her.

About Death

I balanced all, brought all to mind, the years to come seemed waste of breath, a waste of breath the years behind, in balance with this life, this death.

-William Butler Yeats

When giving themselves up to their idea or concept of God, dying people essentially plant seeds that bring forth the possibility of positively moving past their anger.

Initially as such attempts commence the seriously ill or injured person might still show contempt, thinking or uttering phrases like: "Why God? What kind of God would do this to me, a good person? You, God, therefore don't exist. I'm angry with you."

Herein emerges an opportunity to take a long, slow, deep and relaxing breath. Since denial has been obliterated, the person can now strive to use "acceptance of current reality" as achieved in Step 1 to embrace the knowledge that nothing can be changed.

In doing so, the acceptance of and giving one's self up to a higher power becomes a graceful possibility. This stage may take time, particularly if the person's approaching death accelerates. Yet in most cases those still healthy enough to display anger still possess the capability of opening themselves up to their version of the creator.

In doing so, the individual acknowledges and accepts the fact that they are "powerless," just a tiny speck within the entire universe. Giving up their hearts and souls to the higher power invariably can make them mentally stronger, since the concept of God can be all-encompassing and filled with boundless strength or energy.

Even though people may be well known, they hold in their hearts the emotions of a simple person for the moments that are the most important of those we known on earth: birth; marriage; and death.

~ Jackie Kennedy

As the second stage of grief involving anger begins to fade, many people invariably transition into what Kübler-Ross called "bargaining."

Here's where the individual often attempts to make an illogical or fruitless deal with their concept of God or with fate or their perception of the universe.

In this frantic mental bargaining process, which sometimes gets expressed verbally as well, the person ponders promises such as "I'll give up everything I own, if..." or "I'll never sin that way again, if..."

Invariably, lots of people undergoing stage three of the grief process strive to negotiate with the universe for just a few more years of healthy life at the very least.

On a subtle, indirect basis I've seen such "bargaining behavior" many times among the terminally ill or critically injured. Although individuals at this stage might refrain from verbalizing this strategy, their behavior signals an attempt at this method.

I would rather live and love where death is king than have eternal life where love is not.
-Robert Green Ingersoll

Kübler-Ross equated the bargaining process with a person who is about to be divorced by a spouse or left by a lover. The individual realizes that "the end" is near, but strives to buy more time by uttering such phrases as "can we still be friends?"

Sadly, of course, for dying people with incurable diseases or whose ailments have worsened past the point of any hope for recovery, such bargaining fails to get desired results.

To those of us who are healthy, such behavior might seem illogical or a sign that perhaps the person "is going crazy."

Yet to a dying person the bargaining process might seem to make sense. After all, remember as I've indicated earlier,

About Death

Mother Nature has instilled us with an overwhelming and almost unstoppable power and will to survive despite overwhelming odds.

When mindful of such truisms, the display of such bargaining comes into clear view from the eyes of those enjoying vibrant health. Keep in mind that even if you're feeling great today, fast-impending death will eventually happen to you—if you're awake and aware of everything around you as your final moments alive approach.

Which death is preferably to any other? 'The unexpected.'
-Julius Caesar

While engaging in this bargain process, dying people also can begin benefiting mentally by employing the third level of the 12-step strategy.

Here, rather than merely acknowledging a higher power as done in step two, the dying person makes a conscious decision to "turn over their will and their lives" to the higher power, the creator previously accepted in step two.

Just as before, keep in mind that addicts and people obsessed with destructive behaviors have used these strategies with much success.

The ultimate goal here is much different for dying people. Unlike those addicted to alcohol or other substances who want to recover in order to progress into a "better life," dying people realize such an outcome is impossible for them. Eventual death invariably will end life on this earth, at least as we know this experience.

Thus, for the terminally ill or fatally injured individuals, giving up their minds and souls to the higher power might be deemed almost other-worldly.

James W. Forsythe, M.D., H.M.D.

Death not only ends life, it also bestows upon it a silent completeness, snatched from the hazardous flux to which all things human are subject.

-Hannah Arendt

Moving forward, upon transitioning from the stage three bargaining level of grief, many dying people evolve into what Kübler-Ross labeled as "depression."

In this predictable and understandable stage, the terminally ill begin to think that there is no point in bothering with life.

Upon ultimately realizing that the bargaining attempts employed in stage three of grief will fail, the person becomes extremely depressed. Finally, within the mind death has become an unavoidable certainty.

Ensconced in deep depression, dying people overcome by severe sadness often start refusing to see other people. Feeling too depressed to speak and becoming silent, terminally ill people undergoing severe depression sometimes refuse to let friends or relatives visit them.

Such negative progression prevents the dying person from interacting with or connecting with people who want to show them love or to show genuine affection. Kübler-Ross recommended that health care professionals and relatives avoid attempts to make the person happy.

Man is born in a day, and dies in a day, and the thing is easily over; but to have a sick heart for three-fourths of one's lifetime is simply to have death renewed every morning; and life at that price is not worth living.

-Gilbert Parker

On many countless occasions I've interacted with dying people and their families, invariably learning to agree with the suggestions of Kübler-Ross here.

About Death

Mirroring her findings, I also have independently concluded that at least in many instances the depression phase of grief becomes an integral and necessary progression in grieving.

In a sense the extreme depression becomes the body and the mind's "playing out" of life's eventual outcome—death.

This specific type of depression enables the individual to accept the inevitable. Because the mind essentially locks up amid the height of depression, the dying person is allowed to become emotionally detached from the inescapable situation.

Just as Kübler-Ross stated, a vast array of emotions ranging from sadness to uncertainty, fear and regret enable the person to eventually acknowledge his or her current situation.

When the will defies fear, when duty throws the gauntlet down to fate, when honor scorns to compromise with death—that is heroism.
-Robert Green Ingersoll

At this point while easing from the critical and sometimes essential "depression" phase, some dying people who remain cognizant and clear-minded enough can ponder whether additional phases of the 12-step strategy might do them any good at all.

The remaining nine 12-stop phases not previously mentioned range from making a fearless and honest moral inventory of ourselves, to humbly asking God to remove our shortcomings—while also making ourselves ready for the removal of these defects.

Many dying people or their relatives understandably would choose to avoid any type of mental "recovery" strategies. Sometimes such a decision is out of their control.

Decision making obviously becomes unnecessary when the patient dies while locked in denial during the first-phase of the grief process.

Nonetheless when sudden or sooner-than-expected deaths

occur, surviving relatives are often left with their hearts shattered or in a state of mental shock. When this happens getting assistance from a mental health professional or group therapy can help.

Much of the time the urgent and pressing short-term need to handle funeral arrangements initially prevents survivors from entering the intense grief process. Far too often than necessary, I believe, some survivors find themselves suddenly gripped by intense heartache and a sense of loss starting weeks or even months after the death.

For those who seek to understand it, death is a highly creative force. The highest spiritual values of life can originate from the thought and study of death.

-**Elisabeth Kübler-Ross**

A huge percentage of dying people survive long enough to enter what I've personally verified from the initial findings of Kübler-Ross. As she clearly stated in her writings and speeches, the fifth and final stage of the grieving process involves "acceptance."

Well past the phases of denial, anger, bargaining, and depression, when at the last stage the person often thinks and behaves as if fully prepared for the unavoidable.

Although as previously stated numerous times I never tell patients that they should give up or lose hope, lots of the time they begin to accept the fact that they're about to die. These reactions occasionally emerge after various natural remedies or standard treatments have failed to reverse Stage IV cancer's deadly progression.

"Everything will be alright—I know that I'm going to die," becomes a typical statement among many patients at this juncture. "I need to prepare for what will happen."

When this occurs the patient has come to terms with the finality of human life. People destined to become survivors often undergo a similar transition, often focusing their attention on helping to make the dying person as comfortable as possible.

About Death

I've looked at that old scoundrel death in the eye many times but this time I think he has me on the ropes.
- Douglas Macarthur

During the final few weeks of life, dying people occasionally reach and embrace the "acceptance" phase long before their relatives get engulfed in this phase.

The inability, unwillingness or difficulty in dealing with acceptance often impacts surviving people—particularly the parents of small children who died extremely young.

Eternally wise and her teachings spanning the generations, Kübler-Ross expanded her definition of the "death" grief process to include any instance where people suffer the loss of something or someone important to them.

The stages ranging from denial to acceptance impact everyone who strives to understand or to cope with loss. These can include the loss of a job, personal freedom, divorce, formerly large financial holdings, or the breakup with a former lover.

Similar grief stages also sometimes impact people imprisoned for the first time, and individuals striving to cope with a variety of disasters ranging from floods, house fires, catastrophic earthquakes and the eruption of sudden war.

Let us eat and drink neither forgetting death unduly nor remembering it. The Lord hath mercy on whom he will have mercy, etc., and the less we think about it the better.
~ Samuel Butler

While appreciative of the fine work by Kübler-Ross, in a sense I feel as if carrying on today as her halfback in a football game. In a proverbial sense, before her own death she tossed the ball that entails the death process to me and to other medical professionals.

Saddled with this additional responsibility, my job today is to run down the playing field of my professional life in a positive manner. In doing so, I strive to clear a tremendous pathway for many dying people and their families.

Backed by the incredible healing powers of homeopathy and modern medicine, I've been able to identify additional aspects of the grief and dying process.

Today, the issues that face dying and their families often go far beyond the basic challenges confronted by such people during her era. While the overall conclusions of Kübler-Ross remain universal, natural treatments and new medicines sometimes work wonders.

Remember, on occasion treatments that I administer, particularly natural substances, have been known to put cancers in remission among at least some patients who had been considered on "death's doorstep."

We sometimes congratulate ourselves at the moment of waking from a troubled dream; it may be so the moment after death.
                                                                                            -Nathaniel Hawthorne

As stated earlier, as a medical professional I never will—and I never ethically can—give a patient a 100-percent promise that a "cure" is in the offing.

With this understood, there have been numerous times that as a physician and a homeopath I've been able to reverse the conditions of patients once thought terminally ill.

This is not to say, of course, that I or my highly trained clinic staff can "turn off" the cancer switch in patients who have accepted their pending deaths.

A percentage of such patients are far too weak to receive treatments, at a physical stage where the body has evolved well into the process of what doctors call "wasting away." Although only a few exceptions exist, when a person's body weight gets down to "skin and bones" while ravaged by advance-stage diseases including cancer, the person's ability to digest or assimilate vital nutrients has been permanently destroyed.

About Death

Even before they have a chance to visit my office, some patients well into the wasting stage must be told by my clinic staff that there is nothing we can do for them.

Prepare for death if here at night you roam, and sign your will before you sup from home.
-Samuel Johnson

Also as indicated earlier, I have a duty to avoid publishing my patients' names in order to protect their privacy.

Yet I can reveal here without stating their identities that the friends or relatives of numerous world-famous celebrities have been taken them to my clinic while these patients were on the verge of death.

Regrettably, lots of these instances occurred well past the stage of acceptance, past the point where various powerful natural remedies and standard medicine could help.

At this juncture, please remember that I've also previously indicated that other instances involved so-called household names who had been told elsewhere to "get their affairs in order," but got to my office in time for a reversal of the disease.

Additional instances involved movie stars suffering diseases often considered incurable such as pancreatic cancer. I've been told that some ill celebrities wanted to visit my clinic until concerned relatives or friends talked them out of doing so—apparently having the misguided belief that natural medicine is mere "quackery."

Sadly, on numerous occasions my treatments have put specific cancers that once were universally considered death sentences—such as pancreatic cancer—into remission. I'll never know whether my treatments could have saved these famous people who eventually died, after failing to or refusing to visit my clinic.

The only reason I've mentioned these celebrities here is to put the overall situation into perspective. Of course, as human beings these superstars are no different than the rest of us, mere flesh and blood packed with potentially boundless emotions.

I like to behave in an extremely normal, wholesome manner for the most part in my daily life—even if mentally I'm consumed with sick visions of violence, terror, sex and death.

-Courtney Love

Chapter

13

Death-Related Issues Abound

Delving even further than many of the basic findings of Kübler-Ross, I've discovered that as an overall group people who believe their lives have meaning experience less fear during the final few months before death.

As reported in a 2007 book, "A Topical Approach to Life-Span Development," published by McGraw-Hill, studies have borne out this conclusion.

Researchers interviewing 160 people in the final stages before death found less fear among those who reported that they understood the meaning and purpose of their lives.

Conversely, the reports seemed to indicate that people who failed to or refused to acknowledge any meaning in their lives became filled with fear, despair and trepidation amid their final days before dying.

Added to this came the finding that people with religious or intense spiritual belief also tend to experience less fear—while those characteristics also helped them transition quicker out of the denial and depression phases. Later on, I'll discuss more in-depth information on the roles of religion, spirituality and beliefs play in the death process.)

Death, they say, acquits us of all obligations.
-Michel de Montaigne

James W. Forsythe, M.D., H.M.D.

Moving beyond factors involving personal beliefs, some sociologists have equated the grief stages first identified by Kübler-Ross with the basic steps of the human learning process—first identified hundreds or thousands of years ago.

Typically labeled "pedagogy," this term derived from ancient Greek words means "to lead the child." This word signifies how an instructor uses conception and repetition to teach children.

Philosophers, psychologists and educators who embrace the concept of pedagogy believe that pupils instinctively start by mentally ridiculing educational topics, before eventually opposing and then gradually accepting what they've learned.

Numerous philosophers have compared these learning patterns as the equivalent of Kübler-Ross' five grief stages.

Some philosophers claim that dying people mentally behave just like individuals in the learning process where students process various mental patterns in repetition in order to ultimately "learn"—all after initial phases of anger and denial.

Death doesn't affect the living because it has not happened yet. Death doesn't concern the dead because they have ceased to exist.

-W. Somerset Maugham

Some experts have sharply criticized the findings of Kübler-Ross. According to various published reports, George A. Bonanno, a professor of clinical psychology at Colombia University, has tried to develop new strategies for dealing with bereavement and trauma.

Various published articles on Bonanno indicate that his various theories and findings are meant to replace the models regarding grief that are generally accepted today—particularly groundbreaking findings such as those by Kübler-Ross and Sigmund Freud.

Bonanno's various declarations have drawn sharp criticisms.

About Death

The *"Linguia Franca"* has even gone so far as to describe him as "resembling the Grim Reaper, albeit in tanned, rested form."

At least judging by the controversy Bonanno has instilled, his 2010 book may be the biggest groundbreaker on the issue of grief since "On Death and Dying" by Kübler-Ross in 1968. His book rips into the findings of her and others, "The Other Side of Sadness: What the New Science of Bereavement Tells Us About Life After a Loss."

Is Bonanno's attempting to carve new ground, merely as a selfish and misguided attempt to gain attention? Ultimately, the most contentious issue involves his cutting-edge definition of the ability of human beings to become resilient when dealing with loss or trauma.

Some people think football is a matter of life and death. I assure you, it's much more than that.
-Bill Shankly

Reaching a conclusion that I consider mere hype and balderdash, a February 2011 "Scientific American" article quotes Bonanno as arguing that the stages of grief identified by Kübler-Ross simply do not exist.

Is this a misguided, unprofessional attempt on Bonanno's part so that he can fashion himself as being cutting-edge or somehow different?

Well, based on my many thousands of dealings with the death process, I can assure you here that Bonanno's findings are way off the mark—at least in this regard. To pun a well-known phrase, his attentions might be admirable, but his conclusions are "dead wrong."

Without trying to become confrontational or to enter the fray unnecessarily, I still must express my burning need to proclaim that I've personally seen and heard lots of people undergo the stages that Kübler-Ross skillfully identified.

James W. Forsythe, M.D., H.M.D.

If the articles about Bonanno are to be believed, he has concluded that dying or grieving people never actually undergo grief. Instead, he argues that they are "resilient."

Wild animals never kill for sport. Man is the only one for whom the torture and death of his fellow creatures is amusing in itself.

-James Anthony Froude

Despite sharp professional differences between Bonanno and I regarding Kübler-Ross' contributions, there is at least one significant issue upon which we agree.

Like him, I can loudly and affirmatively proclaim that for the most part humans are "highly resilient."

Consistently without any letup whatsoever I've seen instances where terminally ill people and their relatives show seemingly limitless resilience.

Their bodies extremely weak, people considered by medical professionals as "on death's doorstep" sometimes sit up in bed on their last day alive to greet relatives, friends and acquaintances.

The will to live, to retain vibrancy until the very end of life often emerges as a major signal of humanity's strong inner drive to remain resilient from birth until death.

If I die a violent death, as some fear and a few are plotting, I know that the violence will be in the thought and the action of the assassins, not in my dying.

-Indira Gandhi

I've witnessed countless instances where people who have accepted their eventual demise still refuse "to go" until after a long-lost relative shows up to "make peace."

Lots of times this involves putting off death until a favorite or cherished loved one arrives at the deathbed. Additional instances involve situations where relatives "on their way to the deathbed" and the terminally ill person have been estranged or at least ignoring each other for an extended time.

Much of the time for the dying person this intentional delay in death hinges on a burning inner desire to generate some sort of resolution or understanding.

Ultimately, for the dying the overwhelming desire hinges on reaching out emotionally to show love. As our human lives begin to wane we often realize that objects or human possessions literally mean nothing substantial within the great scheme of things in this grand universe.

Instead, the people involved become cognizant of the fact that small disputes or even major conflicts from the past either have or will eventually become pointless, leaving only love, kindness and sympathy in its wake.

What you possess in the world will be found on the day of your death to belong to someone else. But what you are will be yours forever.
-Henry Van Dyke

Sometimes when the dying person holds out for that "long-lost" visitor, closure also comes in the form of at least briefly expressing pent-up anger.

At the start, there's sometimes silence or only a few words exchanged. Pent-up emotions occasionally burst forth in releasing heartache or a sense of regret.

Certainly by this juncture the dying person can barely whisper, too overcome by extreme weakness and final stages of the dying process to effectively communicate.

Medical professionals and relatives of terminally ill people report that the vast majority of instances focus primarily on love, while accepting the current situation.

A miniscule and infrequent rare occurrence involves resentful and extremely angry long-lost or estranged adult children who suddenly arrive in those final days or hours.

"I hate what you have done to me," some angry individuals have been known to mutter to the dying—particularly while the ill person seems to be unconscious. "I'll always be mad at you, and I want you to know how I feel."

I thank my God for graciously granting me the opportunity of learning that death is the key which unlocks the door to our true happiness.
-Wolfgang Amadeus Mozart

The vast majority of us throughout society view any yelling at or vengeful statements to the dying as extremely distasteful and unwarranted.

Without question anyone who treats a dying person in such a hateful tone is thinking only of their own desires and emotions—rather than what the ill person needs.

Such mindless and self-centered emotional displays by physically healthy people serve as an example of the imperfections in our world and in our lives.

Based on my medical experience, I know that chances are strong that much of the time a dying person might seem unconscious—while the mental capacity actually remains clicking in full gear to the final breath.

I believe that lots of the time the dying person fully understands and assimilates everything or at least much of what is said during the final hours of the person's life. Even while seemingly unconscious, the terminally ill might desperately yearn to speak, particularly in response to any harsh statements from unreasonably angry relatives.

About Death

In the attempt to defeat death man has been inevitably obliged to defeat life, for the two are inextricably related. Life moves on to death, and to deny one is to deny the other.

                                                        -Henry Miller

In keeping with the "Lord's Prayer," my senses tell me that emotionally much of the time dying people feel primarily a sense of forgiveness intermixed with love.

At this stage the heart and soul instinctively realize that hate and vengeance ultimately mean very little or nothing.

A warm look in the eyes of dying people, plus the admirable way they strive to hold someone's hand for as long as possible, tells me that they're in the process of melding with and "becoming one" with a loving universe.

One of the most important things that I can teach at this juncture involves love.

Throughout human history some of the world's greatest philosophers, teachers and spiritual leaders including Jesus Christ have taught us that faith, hope and love hail as the greatest gifts bestowed upon human beings.

These factors all play a critical role throughout the various phases of the dying process. Anything regarding "worldly matters" that involves faith and hope seems to transform to the universal, other-worldly or heavenly realm. All along love remains somewhat consistent while also evolving or even growing to new heights.

Death is really a great blessing for humanity; without it there could be no real progress. People who lived forever would not only hamper and discourage the young, but they would themselves lack sufficient stimulus to be creative.

                                                      -Alfred Adler

James W. Forsythe, M.D., H.M.D.

The innate human ability for and propensity for psychological resilience impacts both the dying individual, and also that person's surviving healthy relatives or friends.

In a nutshell, psychologists describe resilience on a psychological level as our ability to cope with emotional and physical stresses.

A key example involves a person immediately after being hit by a car. If the individual remains alive, his adrenaline usually shoots into overdrive.

Particularly in instances where cognitive abilities remain fully functional, the individual's mind initially blasts into orbit—thinking, "Am I going to live? What if anything can I do to remain alive and healthy?"

Remember, as mentioned earlier, a similar situation happened to me when I was a child. After all these years, I've forgotten my exact process from those critical moments. Yet in all likelihood I yearned to do as much as possible to remain alive and healthy after being hit by a car.

Well, in matters of psychological resilience, the same holds true for people when first learning that they have cancer or other fatal afflictions including terminal injuries.

Having a relative who is dying or who has recently died often makes us ponder our own eventual departure from this world—until such time as we return to denial.

Death is the only pure, beautiful conclusion of a great passion.
                                                                    -D.H. Lawrence

At least from my perspective, Bonanno, the Colombia University professor of clinical psychology, seems to discount these deep human emotions.

To me, when developing and eventually proclaiming his controversial theory, Bonanno seems to view human beings as mere animals.

About Death

To imply that dying people never experience denial, anger, bargaining, depression and acceptance is tantamount to categorizing them as mere cows or rodents.

A zebra chased in the African planes by several lions instinctively runs for its life, too caught up in the heat of the moment to experience any semblance of the denial, anger or bargaining. Equally, I believe, a starving gorilla relies on instinct—unable to employ the higher-level emotional and physical options made possible by the superior human IQ.

Our life experiences, particularly interactions with other people and health professionals in a complex and confusing civilization, forces us to face and ponder options and possibilities that wild animals never have to consider.

Not even old age knows how to love death.
-Sophocles

My confusion regarding Bonanno's theory intensified, even after learning that his peer-reviewed research had been conducted during a 20-year span.

Should I believe that this supposed research failed to encounter and chronicle consistent instances where people go into denial when told they are dying?

Why should I embrace a 2010 article in "Time," entitled "New Ways to Think About Grief," describing the conclusion that there are no psychological stages including grief that dying people must or do experience?

My personal observations tell me that such conclusions land far from the bull's-eye. Bonanno's research might be well-intentioned or even admirable, yet as stated earlier my personal interactions with the dying show that Kübler-Ross's findings remain viable.

In essence, at least according to a variety of published reports on Bonanno's findings, most people never grieve when experiencing a loss—but remain resilient, never even coming close to experiencing the five grief stages identified by Kübler-Ross.

If Bonanno actually believes this on a scientific level, then perhaps we as a society should invite him into the rooms of dying people who remain in denial.

What would he say to them?

Perhaps, "You're not in denial, and if you are, that's not part of the grief process."

Bonanno's professional stance becomes the ultimate paradox for dying patients. Everything comes down to the fact that Bonnano is a widely acclaimed professor "denying that dying people are in denial—when, in fact, that's exactly what they are."

Death is one moment, and life is so many of them.
                                                          -Tennessee Williams

Researchers have generated diverse, conflicting conclusions on the issue of whether the findings of Bonanno or Kübler-Ross are on track.

As reported in a 2007 "Journal of the American Medical Association" article, a Yale University study of bereaved people from 2000-2003 generated results consistent with Kübler-Ross's findings.

However, the same "Journal" article notes that some letters subsequently published argued to discount the Kübler-Ross theories, while also criticizing the Yale research.

Joining the fray, according to a 2008 article in "Skeptic Magazine," other mental health professionals also have strived to define as groundless the teachings of Kübler-Ross—most notably the Grief Recovery Institute.

With headquarters in Sherman Oaks, California, the institute strives to disseminate accurate information regarding grief. The institute's Website, GriefRecoveryMethod.com, says that the

About Death

organization was founded by authors of the "Grief Recovery Handbook," John W. James and Russell Friedman.

The leading cause of death among fashion models is falling through street grates.
                                                          -Dave Barry

    The Grief Recovery Institute strives to give accurate details about possible recovery and grief impacting people undergoing all significant emotional losses including divorce and death.
    Mental health professionals say that the ability of people to exhibit psychological resilience enables them to bounce back mentally from disasters or life-changing events.
    The basic separate abilities to cope with typical stresses and the resilience employed to rebound from tragedy are differentiated from a third, but controversial category. This entails changing mentally or "steeling up" following traumatic events.
    Often called "posttraumatic growth" or "steeling effects," such psychological transitions reportedly occur within the psyche of an individual who suddenly gets thrown into a critical situation—such as a war or an accident that simultaneously kills numerous relatives.
    A 2008 article printed by American Psychiatric Publishing describes psychological resilience as not a personal trait, but rather a process that people to undergo due to events—many of those occurrences beyond their control.

Death never takes a wise man by surprise, he is always ready to go.
                                                          -Jean de La Fontaine

    While Bonanno's primary assumptions discounting the findings of Kübler-Ross remain controversial, his declaration regarding the importance of resilience are noteworthy and admirable.

James W. Forsythe, M.D., H.M.D.

His research has enabled many people to better understand that facing death involves much more than merely grief.

The unique ability of humans to generate seemingly unstoppable or relentless resilience can work wonders for the dying and the physically healthy.

Remember those instances previously mentioned where treatments that I administered cured people who literally had been on death's doorstep. Well, in just about every one of those occasions I observed that resilience and a "can-do" attitude played significant roles in enabling those individuals to bounce back physically and mentally.

Most people are fighters by their very nature, particularly those with cancer. Thanks largely to this characteristic the vast majority of my patients have dutifully followed my many suggestions intended for eliminating cancers and eventually enabling them to regain good health.

Man, as long as he lives is immortal. One minute before his death he shall be immortal. But one minute later, God wins.
-
                                                                        -Elie Wiesel

Advanced Stage IV cancer patients primarily show boundless resilient determination in following my orders as their doctor. This remains the case today as I often administer non-poisonous or low-toxic treatments.

Amazingly, the vast majority of my most critical patients from the 1970s into the 1990s displayed similar determination. During that period the only option that I could provide was the poisonous deadly "standard of care" chemotherapy and radiation that mainstream allopathic oncologists are required to follow.

Intense controversy continues to erupt among mental health professionals regarding the impacts and potential psychological assistance that resilience provides in all life issues including severe health problems.

About Death

Some of the hottest topics often under discussion cover everything from how resilience can help adolescents cope with racial discrimination to potentially destructive social value systems. Numerous societies, for instance, teach very young children that killing people of other races or religious beliefs is permissible and even encouraged.

All these factors come to play in a giant, million-piece puzzle when death-related issues emerge. Fear, denial, acceptance and other grief factors often increase or subside within an individual facing death. These mental reactions hinge largely on what the person has been taught, the individual's personal beliefs and even what society expects.

Don't be afraid to feel as angry or as loving as you can, because when you feel nothing, it's just death.
-Lena Horne

The overall issue of psychological resilience coupled with apparent grief stages becomes even more perplexing. These factors become particularly interesting upon realizing that increasing numbers of mental health professionals seem to be questioning the research methodology that Kübler-Ross used.

Numerous published reports in various medical journals in recent years detail the disturbing fact that some current mental health experts have started to discount her methods. The primary complaint here targets the fact that Kübler-Ross developed her findings based on her own personal interviews with dying people.

Medical researchers, doctors and scientists often stress the need to quantify and correlate massive amounts of measurable data when conducting any serious study.

By contrast, at least from the perspective of psychologists who now discount Kübler-Ross' findings, she failed to do critical follow-up interviews with the patients that she interviewed. This woman's critics insist that her efforts should have including the continuous collection of data on each individual until death.

Adding to the controversy, some current researchers even go so far as to suggest that Kübler-Ross should have encouraged or suggested that the patients she interviewed maintain daily diaries chronicling their ongoing emotions.

The nearer people approach old age the closer they return to a semblance of childhood, until the time comes for them to depart this life, again like children, neither tired of living nor aware of death.

-Desiderius Erasmus

As a doctor, I realize the importance and necessity of generating quantifiable data for any and all important scientific research projects. Even so, after a point common sense rather than mere data should rule the day.

To wholly and fully discount Kübler-Ross' findings is tantamount to saying "human beings don't have emotions," or even "what they feel in their hearts does not matter."

I cannot begin to stress this enough. Once again here I feel a critical need to proclaim that "common sense should prevail," especially among those who would sharply criticize the findings of this widely acclaimed late Swiss-American psychiatrist.

Remember, like I have independently done in my own career, Kübler-Ross witnessed thousands of indisputable instances where dying people experience the grief stages she identified.

Streams of other physicians that I've worked with or communicated with at medical conferences have also witnessed these same emotional phases.

Saying that we should be discounted for our basic and irrefutable observations would be tantamount to proclaiming that: "You people are wrong to say that the sun exists, just because you happen to see a bright ball of light in the sky. We need to observe it every day for the rest of your lives in order to us to even begin to believe that the glowing sphere might exist."

About Death

Creativity is not merely the innocent spontaneity of youth and childhood; it also must be married to the passion of the adult human being, which is a passion to live beyond one's death.

-Rollo May

Could some mental health professionals be disclaiming the findings of Kübler-Ross, primarily in order to line their own financial pockets?

Is it possible that huge piles of cash await anyone who develops an "all-new, cutting edge method of dealing with death—an amazing financial windfall?"

For my part, I would never even begin to make such allegations.

To make such a charge would be just as reckless as proclaiming that the findings of Kübler-Ross should be discounted in all instances.

Obviously, people currently dying and their relatives for the most part could care less about any scholarly disputes regarding research methodology. The short-term motivations of these individuals remain impending death.

Sadly, whether or not they realize this, is it possible that those facing death and their relatives are evolving into the potential victims of unscrupulous mental health professionals who proclaim: "we have the best and only answers for you now."

A real hangover is nothing to try out family remedies on. The only cure for a real hangover is death.

-Robert Benchley

Like the vast majority of physicians and mental health experts, my primary concern focuses on the well being of patients.

Rather than solely striving to make the almighty dollar as our only motivation, all doctors need to be wary of anyone who claims to have the "magic cure" for enabling people to mentally cope with death.

With this understood, when asked for my opinion on this critical issue, I urge patients to become weary of anyone who would make such a claim—even by me.

Before seeking the help and guidance of a psychologist or professional grief counselor, you should ask them for their opinions.

Queries such as "What do you think of the findings of Kübler-Ross?" and "what role, if any, do you think psychological resilience plays in helping people to cope?" could help designate a direction that you feel has the greatest potential.

We in the medical profession need to become doubly aware of the ongoing and critical need to help guide patients and their relatives onto beneficial pathways leading to potentially reliable help or guidance.

I went to medical school because I wanted to ask the big questions. Do we have a soul? Does God exist? What happens after death?
-Deepak Chopra

Those of us who acknowledge, understand and appreciate the five grief stages have additional concerns as well.

Just like Kübler-Ross had done, we realize and fully acknowledge the fact that the five grief stages do not always happen in chronological order.

Some of these phases seem to zip past so fast that they're hardly noticeable, adding to the challenge for the dying, their relatives and mental health professionals. Additional occasions might involve instances where a patient gets locked in a particular stage for months or even years.

Yes, like the overall life process, the various stages of the grief are varied and unpredictable in their intensity and overall patterns.

About Death

Perhaps these differences stem from the diverse variances in personalities, the belief systems that people have and how much disease or injury impacts their mental process.

Two soldiers who each are mortally injured in a horrific military aircraft disaster might think and express vastly different emotions until the point of death. One might cry in fear and pain until the bitter end, while the other silently prays to God until his final breath.

I was court martialled in my absence, and sentenced to death in my absence, so I said they could shoot me in my absence.

-Brendan Behan

Through the years I've seen terminal patients of the same gender from similar financial and educational backgrounds react to their pending deaths in sharply different ways. Fear, emotion or negativity motivate some to weep profusely for most of the time that remains, while others spend the bulk of that period choosing to smile or speak cheerily.

The only constant here is that death eventually will occur, something all of us universally share.

Additional challenges also occasionally emerge after the patient or that person's relatives become keenly aware of Kübler-Ross' five grief stages or the various other so-called hot current books such as Bonanno's that primarily focus on resilience.

Kübler-Ross' findings remain so famous that even before receiving news of a malignancy or mortal injuries, some patients and their families are already vaguely or even keenly aware of the five grief stages.

Potential problems might arise in such instances, but potential benefits might blossom as well. A patient recently told that his illness is terminal might become overly anxious or confused by a "one-size-fits-all" declaration of the five grief stages.

James W. Forsythe, M.D., H.M.D.

Madness need not be all breakdown. It may also be breakthrough. It is potential liberation and renewal as well as enslavement and existential death.

- **R.D. Laing**

Judging from my experience, dying people do not universally embrace strange-sounding new information about their health—unless the data offers a potential cure.

A sense of puzzlement and utter bewilderment could very likely emerge when at the onset a terminal patient is told "at this stage, you're supposed to be in denial."

There's a wise old saying that tells us unequivocally that "knowledge is power." Yet being told how and when you should feel a certain way emotionally might fail to impress a dying person as being logical or even meaning with the progression of each new day.

A new danger emerges. Too much information given at an overly rapid rate might spark undue panic and excessive anxiety.

"Am I supposed to feel denial now, or should I start yelling right away to vent my anger?" a patient might proclaim. "All of these emotions, so many of them right now, and I don't truly know what I'm supposed to feel, if anything. So, please leave me alone."

Death be not proud, though some have called thee mighty and dreadful, for thou art not so. For those, whom thou think'st thou dost overthrow. Die not, poor death, nor yet canst thou kill me.

-John Donne

As humans we have much more that we can potentially think about than our ancestors did a mere century ago. Back then, for the most part critically ill patients and their families only knew that they were extremely ill and that death had become a possibility.

About Death

Exacerbating the problem multi-fold during the 1800s and early 1900s, the standard, widely accepted procedures often dictated that a doctor avoid telling a terminal patient that "you are dying." The patient's relatives also were often kept in the dark in this regard.

The confusion grew multi-fold due to the fact at the time the general public remained ignorant or fully unaware of various terminal diseases that today are "common knowledge." Now well into the 21st Century, for instance, most people have a general awareness of many terminal illnesses such as the ultimately fatal amyotrophic lateral sclerosis or ALS, a spinal cord affliction commonly called "Lou Gehrig's Disease."

Today as an overall society we take such knowledge for granted. Yet as recently as the 1920s most people lacked access to reliable information resources necessary to help them identify or even understand serious illnesses or the seriousness of certain traumatic injuries.

For them, that overall situation emerged into a proverbial double-edged sword. Some philosophers have proclaimed that "ignorance is bliss." Certainly a lack of information enabled many people to skirt at least some mental issues.

It is old age, rather than death, that is to be contrasted with life. Old age is life's parody, whereas death transforms life into a destiny; in a way it preserves it by giving it the absolute dimension. Death does away with time.

-**Simone de Beauvoir**

Chapter 14
Technology Issues

The advent of today's rapid-fire, all-encompassing information technology mirrors what the iconic writer Aldous Huxley seemingly predicted at least partly in his classic, timeless 1931 novel, "Brave New World." Considered cutting-edge at the time, the plot focused on issues that seemed far-fetched for that era—everything from considerable advances in reproductive technology to devices that enable people to learn while asleep.

Huxley's conclusions emerged as prophetic, especially when taking into account our overall perceptions of death as viewed by today's technology.

The seemingly unstoppable information super-highway made possible by the Internet has motivated dying people and their relatives to aggressively seek out extensive, detailed information. This, in turn, has generated a proverbial opposite "flip-side" of a coin, as compared to what people faced regarding health and death issues during the first part of the 1900s.

Back then too little information put people in jeopardy, at a time when having more reliable data might have enabled them to seek out and obtain the best cures and remedies.

Today, by contrast people faced with supreme challenges and particularly impending death rush to the Web in an effort to get what they hope will be the best, most critical information. On the negative side, I've seen many instances where incorrect or incomplete data gleaned from the Web gives terminally ill people a false sense of hope or even an undue or unwarranted sense of fatalism.

About Death

Death is the sound of distant thunder at a picnic.
                                                              -W.H. Auden

The terms "pop-psychology" or "fad of the day" sometimes impacts dying people, a direct result of the overload of information available in today's society.

All along, a significant majority of my most-critical, terminal Stage IV cancer patients today are senior citizens—universally the most common age level of people stricken by that severity of the disease.

At least from what I've seen, a relatively large number of these people and their spouses rush to the Internet, making the Web a "be-all, and end-all" solution.

To their great detriment, much of the time these patients and their relatives become confused or angry after initially believing bogus information that they stumble upon. Some of these articles discuss the disease, while others give incorrect details about the dying and grieving process.

Like this or not, doctors need to continually remain prepared for potential verbal disagreements with patients or their relatives rely on incorrect information found on the Web. Based on several instances that I've seen, the recklessly incorrect data found on some Websites gives terminally ill patients and their families a false sense of hope.

Developments such as these, in turn, ultimately can end up locking the psyches of terminally ill patients or their relatives into an unshakable denial phase.

Not the torturer will scare me, nor the body's final fall, nor the barrels of death's rifles, nor the shadows on the wall, nor the night when to the ground the last dim star of pain, is hurled but the blind indifference of a merciless, unfeeling world.

                                                              -Roger Waters

James W. Forsythe, M.D., H.M.D.

Such situations invariably put doctors and many other medical professionals in a precarious situation. In a sense the physician is forced to proverbially "walk on eggshells."

Like trapeze artists striving to traverse high-strung tight-ropes, doctors occasionally find themselves having to delicately or even directly explain that certain information gleaned from the Web is "wrong," and that death remains imminent.

When this happens, the patient or that person's relatives might become unduly angry at the doctor, thereby delving—perhaps unnecessarily—into one of the five critical grief stages.

All along, the situation becomes increasingly paradoxical, because today's information super-highway also occasionally enables dying or seriously ill patients to determine that their doctor is "wrong" or that "other more viable strategies exist."

As a prime example, here I'm motivated to mention my numerous other books that have enabled terminal or seriously ill patients to learn that there often is a better way thanks largely to effective non-toxic treatments that I or other homeopaths can provide.

Please remember, as previously mentioned, there have been instances where doctors elsewhere have told certain patients to "get your affairs in order"—before those individuals visited my clinic, only to be cured.

In every death a busy world comes to an end.
-Mason Cooley

There has been an apparent increase in recent years of instances where "false-positive" results have generated an incorrect, false diagnosis of a "death-sentence"-level cancer. Thanks partly to advances in modern medicine, new treatments often eradicate diseases once believed always terminal.

Practitioners of natural or homeopathic medicines also occasionally prove such diagnosis as wrong. Professionals

About Death

of natural medicines including homeopaths occasionally use treatments that are thousands of years old to lengthen the life expectancies of patients once deemed by modern medicine as "beyond hope" for a cure.

Collectively and individually, these positive factors serve as my primary motivation for never telling my own patients to "get their affairs in order."

Does this mean that I'm locked in denial, just like a terminally ill person experiencing the first stage of grief?

Does my positive, can-do attitude serve as a way for me to express my anger against the mainstream medical industry—which forces most Stage IV cancer patients to endure deadly radiation or chemo?

To the contrary, I choose to avoid telling most patients that "you are going to die," simply because the vast majority of these people need to remain open to the possibility of a last-minute cure when already under my care.

Once you accept your own death, all of a sudden you're free to live. You no longer care about your reputation. You no longer care except so far as your life can be used tactically to promote a cause you believe in.
                                                                -Saul Alinsky

Chapter 15

Apparent "Life After Death"

"**D**octor, I died last night, and then came back to life," some patients have told me.

My interactions with people who insisted they had such experiences began in the early 1970s, shortly before the 1975 publication of Ray Moody's bestseller "Life After Life"—followed by a steady succession of other successful books on the topic by other authors.

The individual stories of my patients who reported such experiences varied somewhat. Some basic themes or occurrences involving these events remained common among them all.

Middle-aged and elderly patients who claimed to have undergone such experiences invariably spoke of bright lights. Some described heading toward a bright beam near the end of a tunnel.

Almost all of them recounted vivid stories of being met by a person or "spirit," usually someone they knew who had previously died. The specific settings and characters varied in these tales.

It is impossible that anything so natural, so necessary, and so universal as death, should ever have been designed by providence as an evil to mankind.
                                                            -Jonathan Swift

In each instance I made no attempt to discount their stories, or to tell these people that "what you think occurred never possibly could have happened."

About Death

All these individuals claimed that their experiences were "real." Perhaps most of all, they recalled overwhelming sensations of peace, tranquility and love.

Much of the time, these individuals reported that they did not want to return to their current bodies, to "come back to life."

Although a God-loving, God-fearing Christian, my job as a medical professional dictates that I avoid attempting to serve as a Biblical preacher or a spiritual counselor.

Without telling my patients this, I personally believed that there was a strong probability that perhaps all or at least some of what they claimed actually happened.

The common factors in their stories led me to think that "perhaps there is something really interesting going on here."

A man may devote himself to death and destruction to save a nation; but no nation will devote itself to death and destruction to save mankind.
-Samuel Taylor Coleridge

I made no attempts to scientifically study their after-life claims, instead focusing on enabling these patients to recover or to lessen their negative physical symptoms.

Thus, my opinion regarding the believability of their tales was not based on sound, verifiable science, but rather on my consistent personal observations of their stories.

Increasing numbers of scientists in recent years have discounted all such claims of visiting the afterlife. Those complaining from the scientific community insisted that the bright lights and the sense of peace that the dying claimed to have experienced were merely the natural predictable biological reactions within the brain.

The resulting disputes intensified between these scientists and believers of the after-life. Until the release of the book you are reading now, I have chosen to remain silent on the issue, preferring to focus my attention on medicine rather than theology or spiritualism.

James W. Forsythe, M.D., H.M.D.

As far as I can tell no one on either side of this issue "can prove scientifically beyond a shadow of a doubt if the after-life exists or does not exist."

Once you start doing only what you've already proven you can do, you're on the road to death.
-Jerry Seinfeld

Certainly my declaration of personally believing that the after-life exists will bring great hope to at least some terminally ill patients.

Yet at least when within the confines of our limited, non-spiritual world I'm in the same boat as all other scientists or doctors who lack the ability to prove this point.

From the perspective of scientists, just saying that you believe something does not necessarily make that opinion true.

Conversely, from the religious or spiritual perspective, the failure of scientists to believe in God or the after-life could very well prevent them from knowing "the truth."

Adding complexity to the situation, patients who claim that they've already visited the after-life insist that what they saw, felt, smelled and experienced during those treks was "as real as real can possibly be."

From the perspective of many people who strongly believe in God, any attempt to discount such tales of the after-life is tantamount to sacrilegious. Many religious people proclaim that to discount the word of God is sinful, wicked and even evil.

Don't be afraid of death so much as an inadequate life.
-Bertolt Brecht

The late legendary singer Lou Rawls, a multi-platinum recording artist whose 60 albums sold more than 40 million units, once told a journalist about the entertainer's after-life experience.

Rawls recalled being knocked unconscious when a passenger in a car early in his recording career in the late 1950s. Rawls told of floating above his own body during an ambulance ride to the hospital. The singer also vividly remembered floating near the ceiling of the hospital emergency room, looking down at doctors as they worked to restart his heart.

While that was going on, Rawls said, his spirit was pulled upward through a tunnel toward a bright light. Once finally inside a heavenly place Rawls was met by the glowing, love-filled spirits of deceased relatives.

The entertainer also remembered talking briefly with Our Creator, who spoke of the importance of boundless, eternal love. The next thing that Rawls could remember was of awakening in the hospital recovery room.

From that point forward Rawls strived to emit the essence of pure, uncensored love in his own voice—particularly during his successful solo presentations. The singer credited much of his professional success on the lessons given by the Lord in the afterlife.

The human consciousness is really homogenous. There is no complete forgetting even in death.

- D.H. Lawrence

Such brief forays into the after-world often are called "near-death experiences" or NDE. Volumes of published news reports, magazine articles and books list other common attributes reported by people who claim to have experienced this phenomenon.

Besides sensations of being detached from their bodies and feeling as if their spirits are levitating, people who nearly died often report having experienced a sense of warmness and complete serenity.

At least while undergoing an NDE, these people say, that they feel no fear whatsoever when suddenly seeing the mysterious light—which invariably seems to emit the essence of eternal, boundless and universal love.

Lots of people who have made such claims report that they were pronounced clinically dead, before either naturally reawakening on their own or being revived by medical professionals such as doctors or paramedics.

Recent news articles have reported that the instance of NDEs has increased along with advancements that have increased the ability of medical professionals to revive patients whose hearts and breathing have stopped.

Take care of your life and the Lord will take care of your death.
                                                              -George Whitfield

As previously indicated, some medical professionals and scientists have discounted the stories of such patients as merely hallucinations.

This has failed to stop a number of religious believers, practitioners of parapsychology and even some scientists from proclaiming that the common links told in these stories should be considered as profound.

The information, they say, is strong and consistent enough to signify the existence of an after-life or at the very least evidence that a "mind-body dualism" exists.

This philosophy embraces the duality between the mind and the body, which both together and individually are equally joined with all matter throughout the universe.

Thousands of years ago the Greek philosophers Aristotle and Plato, embraced this concept of multiple, dully joined souls.

From their view, when translated in a manner that today's everyday people can understand, these dualities also are tied to the characteristics and functions of other people, plants and animals.

All these attributes are broken down into subsets. A key example involves people and animals, which collectively share yearnings for such things as food.

About Death

Just as I shall select my ship when I'm about to go on a voyage, or my house when I propose to take a residence, so I shall choose my death when I am about to depart from life.
-Seneca

Many hundreds of years after Plato and Aristotle, during the 1600s the philosopher René Descartes also championed the concept of dualism. He clearly defined and identified the mind as a non-physical substance, separate from the body and the brain—although dependant on that organ while alive.

All along, the mind as defined by Descartes also possessed or controlled the ability of human beings to become uniquely conscious of their own existence.

Even today these factors are important to consider when reviewing or arguing about the possibility of whether near-death experiences and the after-life actually exist.

Although they sharply disagree on this issue, many on both sides of the controversy seem to agree that this dualism impacts everything from our priorities regarding the importance of physical items to our very belief systems.

Nevertheless, as reported in numerous philosophical and medical journals, modern science still has failed to find conclusive evidence to support dualism.

Instead, some intellectuals prefer to embrace yet another philosophical belief system, a theory called "physicalism"—which insists that only physical things exist. Austrian philosopher, political economist and sociologist Otto Neurath first coined this phrase in the early 20th Century.

Like all of us in this storm between birth and death, I can wreak no great changes on the world, only small changes for the better, I hope, in the lives of those I love.
-Dean Koontz

James W. Forsythe, M.D., H.M.D.

Side-stepping the issue of whether what people report seeing, hearing and feeling during NDEs are "true," articles published as recently as 2013 quote various philosophers and scientists as insisting that such experiences cannot be considered as merely "imagined."

Instead, these people argue, the physiology of the individual reporting an NDE could cause them to believe that they had "lived" through something that was not "reality."

Admittedly only people with fairly high IQs and conceptual vision are deemed qualified to fully understand and mentally grasp the complex interweaving of these terminologies and explanations.

Ultimately, for many of today's common, average, everyday people the question remains: "Do near-death experiences and the after-life actually exist."

For people currently diagnosed as terminal and their families, these complexities and integral sciences mean very little. Particularly among those lacking religious faith, all they know for sure is that pending death is currently looking at them straight in the eye.

It is natural to indulge in the illusions of hope. We are apt to shut our eyes to that siren until she allures us to our death.
-Gertrude Stein

The concept and belief in near-death experiences are so widespread and generally accepted that nearly eight million Americans report that they have experienced NDEs, according to results of a nationwide Gallup Poll.

Even if an extremely small percentage of these people actually experienced an NDE, the totals are significant and worthy of attention.

To wholly discount such claims without giving the situation at least some amount of serious study would be a slap in the face to the general public and even the concept of science.

About Death

In fact, according to an article in the "Journal of Advanced Nursing," estimates on the number of people who've undergone such experiences may actually be underestimated.

Such claims have generated so much attention that the phenomenon of NDEs is now being studied by psychologists, psychiatrists and practitioners of hospital medicine.

Nothing endears so much a friend as sorrow for his death. The pleasure of his company has not so powerful an influence.

-David Hume

Contrary to popular belief, the reports of NDEs and the similarities of such "after-death" travels are far from new.

As far back as 400 years before the birth of Jesus Christ, people reported undergoing such experiences—as reported in the iconic, still-world-famous "Plato's Republic."

Plato described the revelations or declarations of soldiers who initially seemed to have died, only to later be revived by their comrades or naturally reawakening.

More than 2,000 years after Plato in the 1890s, the French epidemiologist Victor Egger paved the way for today's modern NDE research. Egger generated the term "experience of imminent death" following various discussions among physiologists and philosophers.

The concept never catapulted into the widespread public mindset until 1975 when Moody's blockbuster mentioned earlier enjoyed explosive worldwide sales.

Life and death are important. Don't suffer them in vain.

-Bodhidharma

Critics seized upon the seemingly unstoppable public craze as steadily increasing numbers of people across many countries learned of near-death experiences.

James W. Forsythe, M.D., H.M.D.

Although reports of NDEs had common features such as meeting dead relatives and "seeing God," critics noted that each person making such a claim invariably described experiencing religious beliefs and cultural aspects prevalent within their own societies.

People worldwide do not universally report "seeing Christ." For instance, people reporting NDEs from some countries say that encountered Buddha while others saw other gods. The deity revered most frequently in the person's society often prevails.

Such apparent consistencies that vary among cultures eventually become psychological fodder or scientific weaponry among those who discount the validity such stories.

Besides the attributes mentioned earlier, many of those experiencing NDEs report: sensations of seeing or feeling they're outside their bodies; a tunnel that leads to the light; receiving a review of their entire lives; and occasionally previews of their future lives.

If Shaw and Einstein couldn't beat death, what chance have I got? Practically none.
                                                                    - Mel Brooks

One of the most interesting aspects that intrigue many people hearing these details involves the "life review" process. Within the span of a few seconds, some people who experienced NDEs say, they reviewed much or all of their entire lives.

Lots of these stories involve a review of in-depth and highly detailed information assimilated in chronological order.

Some observers equate this unique and mysterious process with the age-old saying of having their "live flash before their eyes."

Besides Moody, other scholars chronicling and studying the NDE survivors' tales about life review include Kenneth Ring, a University of Connecticut professor emeritus specializing in psychology, founding editor of the "Journal of Near-Death Studies."

About Death

Another pivotal researcher playing as significant role in giving the public intriguing details about NDEs has been Barbara Rommer, author of the 2000 book "Blessing in Disguise: Another Side of the Near Death Experience."

As reported by Rommer, about 17 percent of NDEs were distressing and extremely frightening to the people who experienced them. If true, this means that nearly one out of every five NDEs involve people who experience hellish visions in the after-life.

Well, to the people who pray for me to not only have an agonizing death, but then be reborn to have an agonizing and horrible eternal life of torture, I say, "Well, good on you. See you there."

-Christopher Hitchens

According to Rommer's book, she interviewed 300 people who experienced hellish NDEs. Some of these individuals had undergone harsh reviews of their current lives. Adding unexpected intrigue to the already mysterious situation, at least by Rommer's account many of these people developed psychic or healing powers after "from the dead."

Should we discount such tales as pure nonsense, virtually impossible?

Or, as some believe, are these reports real? Is the Lord, Creator or God giving a message to those NDE survivors about the importance of love, and ultimately to us as well?

Taking this pathway even further, another question arises: How much should currently healthy people and terminally ill individuals strive to ponder such situations?

For those of us who believe in God while also giving the concept of NDEs credence, the obvious answer becomes straightforward: "Show other people in this world as much love and kindness as we can, while we still have time."

James W. Forsythe, M.D., H.M.D.

Death obsesses me, yes it does. I can't really understand why it doesn't obsess everyone—I think it does really, I'm just a little more out about it.
-J.K. Rowling

Obviously to pun a phrase, "scared to death" following their hellish NDEs, some survivors interviewed by Rommer quickly changed their lives around. Numerous instances involved removing negative behaviors once used in the past, stopping destructive habits, and even changing careers in order to take a more positive and loving pathway through the remainder of life.

Rommer's book noted that many negative-NDE sufferers that she interviewed had attempted suicide or had expressed hateful, harmful or extremely distressful feelings toward others earlier prior to their hellish near-death experiences.

In Rommer's book and throughout many other articles describing life reviews during NDEs, many people who experienced them remember doing so in the presence of non-human, "otherworldly" beings.

If true, could these have been angels of the Lord or perhaps even saints?

Just as intriguing emerges the question of whether each of us invariably enter situations where we must openly and honestly review our own lives.

For thousands of years various religions have proclaimed that each and every one of us will eventually have to undergo a "judgment day."

Success is like death. The more successful you become, the higher the houses in the hills get and the higher the fences get.
-Kevin Spacey

Lots of NDE veterans, of both the heavenly and the hellish varieties, have reported that the "otherworldly beings" present during life-reviews weren't passing judgment.

Instead, NDE survivors said they seized upon a sense of responsibility to judge themselves during the life reviews, harshly in some instances.

Psychologists and paranormal researchers also have extensively detailed instances where people have suddenly reviewed and judged their entire lives while undergoing extreme physical danger—not just during NDEs.

Instances where life reviews occur after the heart has stopped almost always involve a "view" or perspective far different than that typically experienced while alive as a human being. Some NDE survivors insist that their journey was in a three-dimensional or holographic sense—and sometimes even panoramic in nature.

Perhaps most intensely, at least as reported by a vast majority of these people, the temporarily dead person's perception throughout an NDE is extremely vivid.

Amid her own life-review, at least one person said, she viewed her life on earth thus far as a vision of hell itself.

Do not seek death. Death will find you. But seek the road which makes death a fulfillment.
- **Dag Hammarskjold**

In a bestselling account of her own near-death experience, Betty Eadie won praise for her vivid descriptions.

The runaway sales of her "Embraced by the Light" in 1992 were followed by additional successes of "The Awakening Heart" in 1996, "The Ripple Effect" in 1999, and "Embraced by the Light: Prayers and Devotions for Daily Living" in 2001.

The continued success of Eadie's books and others on this topic by additional authors signifies that the public still has a desperate craving to know what will happen to each of us after we die.

James W. Forsythe, M.D., H.M.D.

At my clinic the inquisitive look in the eyes of many patients indicates that perhaps many of them have similar curiosity although—as previously indicated—we rarely speak about death and particularly anything that might occur to their souls afterward.

Many of them, particularly those eventually deemed terminal, might find at least some solace in Eadie's books, particularly "Embraced by the Light." The author vividly describes her unique NDE while recovering from surgery in 1973 at age 31.

All societies on the verge of death are masculine. A society can survive with only one man; no society will survive a shortage of women.
-Germaine Greer

Eadie remembered initially feeling lifeless before hearing a "pop" sound accompanied by an immediate sense of release from her body.

Suddenly engulfed by a sense of freedom, she began moving about freely without being slowed or hindered by gravity and inertia.

Three angelic beings soon met Eadie, who remembers them mentioning her previous existences. If true, could those have been indications of a reincarnation process, or were her memories at least in this regard mere fantasy?

The author's vivid and highly descriptive writings give intrinsic and compelling detail of her traveling to various terrestrial locations. These sites included her home; all sites were visited instantaneously merely by thinking about them.

She then started returning to the hospital, only to immediately find herself in a tunnel. There, Eadie says, she encountered other spirits, beings or entities. She got an immediate sense that these beings were undergoing some sort of transition.

About Death

I saw also that there was an ocean of darkness and death, but an infinite ocean of light and love, which flowed over the ocean of darkness.
-George Fox

Initially approaching intense light while traveling through the tunnel, Eadie entered a place she described as heaven immediately before being embraced by Jesus Christ.

From this point her writings chronicling the experience cover a wide range of topics that had not yet been broached by other reports of NDEs. Her additional subjects covered everything from specific descriptions about prayer to how life was created.

If Eadie's account is true, various "beings" in the afterworld took her to a "library of knowledge," where she was able to review all of human history. The intrigue becomes doubly intense when considering the potentialy validity of her additional reports claiming that she was allowed to visit or observe life on distant planets.

Eadie remembers learning that she would have to return to her earthly body, told that she had died prematurely and would be revived. Various published accounts indicate that Eadie's physician later verified that her vital signs had stopped during a nurses' shift change.

Needless to say, Eadie's first book and her subsequent publications fueled increasingly intense public interest about NDEs. The topic likely will continue sparking curiosity, particularly if and when scientists generate irrefutable evidence, either supporting or disclaiming such reports.

The call of death is a call of love. Death can be sweet if we answer it in the affirmative, if we accept it as one of the great eternal forms of life and transformation.
-Herman Hesse

James W. Forsythe, M.D., H.M.D.

The fairly steady, strong sales of such books indicate to me that terminally ill people and anyone intrigued by death can easily get magnetized by the positive possibilities that NDEs seem to signify.

Perhaps one of the most compelling factors sparks the imagination, the many reported instances where those surviving these experiences insist that they were taught or discovered intricate details regarding the nature of the universe.

Throughout human history people have strived to discover and find the very essence of their lives, why they exist and particularly why each of us eventually has to die. Besides what various religions tell us, the reports of NDEs provide a way to review potential answers.

In fact, these sensations become so satisfying to the majority of NDE survivors that they almost always independently report in essence that: "I became depressed at the thought of returning back to this earthly life."

For terminally ill people such statements might ignite potential hope, but only if they choose to believe such a sensational transition awaits them—made possible only by their own deaths.

What is the value of sticking a microphone in a man's face right after he has learned of his wife's death?
                                                              -Jessica Savitch

Some researchers have thoroughly scoured interviews with NDE survivors, indicating that nearly two-thirds of them reported strong feelings of peace and contentment. Published accounts indicate that Kenneth Ring, the University of Connecticut professor emeritus, found that from among the total individuals interviewed, only about 10 per eventually "entered the light."

However, as indicated earlier, differences in NDE reports that vary among cultures has provided an extensive opportunity to question the validity of such stories.

About Death

This might be countered at least somewhat by tales such as that of Eadie, who reports she was told during her NDE that God has a purpose for enabling people to worship in different religions—marked with separate levels of spiritual enlightenment.

Such arguments fail to sway those who insist that the gullible public should never believe such tales, which the opponents of NDE describe as outlandish.

Sparking additional concerns and counter-claims, Eadie remembers being told during her NDE that reincarnation simply does not exist—that each of us only has one life.

His death was the first time that Ed Wynn ever made anyone sad.
                                                              -Red Skelton

Besides rattling people who embrace the concept or belief of reincarnation, Eadie also insists that she learned during her NDE that God and Jesus Christ are not "one and the same"—a concept in sharp contrast to the teachings of Christianity.

Adding fuel to the proverbial fire, many of those who insist that NDEs actually occur including Eadie say that although humans have been given "free-will" in order to give them opportunities for doing good things or making mistakes—"there are no accidents."

Once again, we have instances where life and eventually death seem to make little sense at least when thoroughly analyzed based on statements by NDE survivors.

Increasingly determined to verify the viability, believability and possibility of NDE claims—or the lack of such apparent events—neuroscientists have begun to study these reports and interview survivors.

Hopefully, such efforts will someday reach a definitive, undisputable conclusion on whether NDEs actually exist. Neuroscience is deemed the best possible field of study to ultimately determine the validity of such claims, delving into the interaction between the brain with the body's neural systems that impact everything from memory to emotions.

The acceptance of death gives you more of a stake in life, in living life happily, as it should be lived—living for the moment.

-Sting

Vowing to generate conclusive answers, those intrigued with or inspired by NDEs have formed a non-profit organization, the International Association for Near Death Studies, based in Durham, North Carolina.

Numerous researchers including authors of books about NDEs first formed the association way back in 1981, when the organization's original name was "The Association for the Scientific Study of Near-Death Phenomenon." It started in Connecticut where professor Ring was based, but later moved to North Carolina.

The association's notable responsibilities include the ongoing publication of "The Journal of Near-Death Studies."

Once called "Anabiosis," the academic journal continues as a quarterly peer-reviewed publication. For more information on the journal, visit iands.org.

The wide variety of topics covered during the journal's first three decades range from how people can adjust and accept their return to life following an NDE to the role such apparent events play in the evolution of the human consciousness, and similarities with experiences using psychedelic drugs.

An important consequence of freeing oneself from the fear of death is a radical opening to spirituality of a universal and non-denominational type.

-Stanislav Grof

About Death

As a physician and a homeopath specializing in standard medicines and natural treatments for a variety of diseases—particularly cancer, I have no specific recommendation on whether terminally ill people should study NDE reports.

Remember, as a doctor I avoid serving as an official spiritual or religious counselor, and other physicians should not be expected to do so.

At least based on my research, I have been unable to find any in-depth, long-term and intense research on whether introducing the concept of NDEs to the terminally ill ultimately helps them cope mentally with grief and worries about their pending deaths.

Nonetheless, with help from their families and friends, or perhaps on their own, some of these people might feel a need to seize upon this option—to at the very least investigate the possibilities of what may occur.

Right away upon initially getting their diagnosis of a malignancy, some patients obviously feel sad or doomed at least at the onset. Tales such as those provided by NDE reports might tend to make them lean at least somewhat emotionally in quite the opposite direction—as if there's a possibility that they're about to be "set free."

Loved. You can't use it in the past tense. Death does not stop that love at all.
-Ken Kesey

Chapter 16

Religion and Philosophy Enter the Equation

Stories similar to those of entertainer Lou Rawls' and other NDE survivors have steadily emitted into the general mainstream news media in recent years. Best-selling books on the subject have separately chronicled such after-life stories as the near-death of a preacher's child following surgery and the near-drowning of a doctor in a boating accident.

In all likelihood huge sections of the public desperately yearn for true-life, real stories such as these.

People everywhere instinctively yearn for real-life proof that their experiences are not limited to the brief time each of us has during a single lifetime here on earth.

Atheists and agnostics discount such yearnings as pure foolishness. These people generally insist that our bodies lack souls. They think that when we die "that's it."

Such prognosticators are in a tiny minority of the entire world population.

For thousands of years the vast majority of people in the civilized world have religion or spiritual beliefs that universally give hope for an afterlife.

Sleep is good, death is better; but of course the best thing would to have never been born at all.
-Heinrich Heine

About Death

For Buddhists, the life and death cycle continues at a relentless pace until such time as the soul finally achieves nirvana—after which there is no life at all.

The bulk of other religions promise eternal life in the afterworld or heaven, primarily for those who "obey God's laws while here on earth."

The many versions of the afterlife are so diverse and complex that sociologists insist that this concept impacts everything from religion and mythology to philosophy and fiction.

Depending largely on the socially acceptable belief systems where they live, overall the 7 billion people now living worldwide have many afterlife options to consider.

As opposed to the atheist definition of "eternal oblivion" after death, some of the other philosophies or belief systems center on "naturalism." This philosophy or belief system insists that nothing exists beyond our natural world—as dictated by and mandated by the laws of nature.

Naturalism confines itself to chemical and physical laws that are generally accepted and agreed upon by today's scientists. People embracing this belief argue that spirits ghosts and religious deities simply do not exist, because the natural universe lacks any purpose for or use for them.

Creation destroys as it goes, throws down one tree for the rise of another. But ideal mankind would abolish death, multiply itself million upon million, rear up city upon city, save every parasite alive, until the accumulation of mere existence is swollen to a horror.

-D.H. Lawrence

The complexity of the issue becomes even more intriguing when taking into account the beliefs of people called "pantheists." Although embracing science, these individuals insist that the natural universe or nature is "one in the same" with God.

The after-life concept seems to become doubly confusing

here. Depending on their own particular beliefs and scientific conclusions, some pantheists even go so far as to insist that nature was created by one or more gods.

The push toward naturalism became so intense during the 1900s that some intellectuals even began insisting that all philosophy should be based on scientific methods.

Thus, the opportunity for continued conflict strengthened and intensified among scientists and standard theologians, particularly regarding issues involving the afterlife.

While some of them flat-out discount the possibility of heaven or the afterlife, some practitioners of naturalism say that their belief system stretches back thousands of years—well before many of today's religions or belief systems began.

We want our idols to be dead because it makes death a less scary place.
-Doug Coupland

On the flip side of naturalism, the vast majority of the world embraces religions or spiritual beliefs that delve into what theologians call the "supernatural."

These are entities such as God, Jesus Christ and Buddha, none of them subject to the known scientific laws of physics.

Experts in theology and in human belief systems tell us that the definition of supernatural goes beyond religion, covering any "perceived" or "believed" occurrences that seem to defy the known and agreed-upon laws of physics.

While many people who devote their lives to religion might yearn to say otherwise, supposed supernatural processes that seemingly defy physics include events deemed as "paranormal" or even claims and beliefs involving "occultism" or "spiritualism."

For some terminally ill people and their families, particularly those not already familiar with these belief systems, the possibilities might seem overwhelming.

About Death

By many accounts numerous dying people, particularly those engulfed in the "bargaining" phase of grief described by Kübler-Ross, will try to believe just about anything if they think that doing so will spare them from death.

Families survive, one way or another. You have a tie, a connection that exists long after death through many lifetimes.
-Jessica Lange

For as long as their mental faculties still permit, dying people who have already believed in the teachings of their churches or religions often have somewhere to turn for guidance and for solace—their personal faith.

Yet many times I've seen instances where the inescapable situation of becoming "terminal" quickly tests the faith that an individual once profoundly had.

"Why is God doing this to me?" a dying person who grew up steeped in religion might say angrily. "If there really is a God, why does he do bad things to good people like me? In fact, I don't think any more that there can be a God."

Such reactions seem predictable and maybe even understandable, particularly among observers who view Kübler-Ross's five-stages of grief with at least some degree of validity. Carrying forward with the patterns already mentioned the news of malignancy might also test the faith of the terminally ill person's relatives and friends.

When interacting with people undergoing this critical juncture in the life-transition process, the latest supposed cool thing to say is that "everything happens for a reason" and that "this must be part of the Lord's grand plan—which we aren't meant to understand."

James W. Forsythe, M.D., H.M.D.

The ideal death, I think, is what was the ideal Victorian death, you know, with your grandchildren around you, a bit of sobbing. And you say goodbye to your loved ones, making certain that one of them has been left behind to look after the shop.

-Terry Pratchett

Statements about life's supposed "grand plan" as previously mapped out by God obviously make little sense at least to some dying people.

Remember, as stated earlier for thousands of years people have looked to their religions for guidance in developing personal faith for understanding why death ultimately will take them from this world.

Some believers in the Lord Jesus Christ, particularly Catholics, look to a variety of supernatural events chronicled in the Bible as a basis for their faith. These include beatific visions such as gazing upon or conversing with heavenly angels or the Virgin Mary, the mother of Jesus.

Many of today's most learned, scholarly scientists will say that there is no scientific, evidence proving that such events occurred. Yet for the people who believe, such events intensify their feelings for—and their reasoning—in holding faith.

Such beliefs, in turn, can emerge as formidable tools in helping terminally ill people and their relatives get a sense that they're able to mentally cope with the pending death.

Death is the mother of Beauty; hence from her, alone, shall come fulfillment to our dreams and our desires.

-Wallace Stevens

Lots of dying people and their relatives suddenly "find God" when the Grim Reaper fast approaches. Far more times than I possibly could remember in full detail, I've seen instances where these individuals scurried back to the church as soon as death started rushing toward them.

Rather than being judgmental on my part, this is just a basic observation that I feel a need to report. This way, many people can enable themselves to get a better sense of focus, depending on their faith—perhaps ultimately deciding to visit representatives of their church for spiritual guidance.

Much of the time physically healthy relatives of the terminally ill—often people who have not attended church for many decades--rush into an "emergency mode."

Struck by a suddenly profound sense of urgency these people summon preachers or priests to perform various types of last rites sanctioned by various religions.

Rather than call them "hypocrites," let us say that these individuals are merely doing their best to enable themselves and the dying to cope. People from countless cultures have behaved in similar ways for thousands of years.

My mortal foe can no ways wish me a greater harm than England's hate; neither should death be less welcome unto me than such a mishap betide me.
                                                            -Queen Elizabeth I

Many churches and religious beliefs seek to condemn or even to ridicule anyone who might dare to criticize or to vilify their supernatural beliefs.

Particularly in religious matters that involve death, those who would dare question the church's miracles or beliefs about death get labeled as heretics, infidels or blasphemers.

"If the church says it must be so, then I believe that I will go to heaven when I die if I ask forgiveness for my sins," a dying person might say. "God, accept me into your loving and giving hands, for I'm ready to go into your eternally loving arms."

Such statements make perfect sense to me and to streams of

other professionals including doctors and nurses.

Although many of us never embrace any particular religion or belief system, through observation over a period of years people serving in the medical industry have witnessed the boundless power that faith can give to dying people and their families.

Generosity during life is a very different thing from generosity during the hour of death; one proceeds from genuine liberality and benevolence, the other from pride or fear.

-Horace Mann

The Biblical teachings of Jesus raising Lazarus from the dead, and of the Virgin Mary giving birth without having intimate relations with a man, are just a few of the supernatural stories that can help give at least some comfort to dying Christians.

Besides so-called mainstream religions such as Christianity and Judaism, other belief systems that describe the afterlife are esotericism and metaphysics. Many volumes that fill entire libraries have been written on these complex, highly detailed topics.

In essence, esotericism—sometimes called "spirituality"—is deemed by much of society as an opinion or as a belief system. Sometimes the various forms of esotericism are tied to philosophies developed by people, or spin-offs from traditional religions.

Often dealing at least partly with how people should cope with or deal with death, these entail a massive spectrum of religious movements and philosophies.

Frequently shunned by mainstream religions that consider them "evil" or "the devil's work," these include everything from astrology and alchemy to Christian mysticism and Freemasonry. Many of these esoteric philosophies and religious movements focus largely on generating a sense of meaning and belief from the writings or symbols originally derived from mainstream religions.

About Death

The meaning of life is not to be discovered only after death in some hidden, mysterious realm; on the contrary it can be found by eating the succulent fruit of the Tree of Life and by living in the here and now as fully and creatively as we can.
                                                            -Paul Kurtz

Many people who embrace beliefs and philosophies within the esoteric realm concentrate at least partly on how their beliefs interact with death. They also focus much of their attention on symbolism or the specific meaning of historic religious texts.

As described by Plato long before Christ, the term "eso" designates the quest to find "inner things," while also using to phrase "exo" in describing "outside things." The philosopher Aristotle subsequently made note of these distinctions.

Without attempting to get overly intellectual about the importance of the esoteric process, I still sense an urgent need to stress the fact here that dying people often strive to find some sort of meaning in their lives.

Particularly in instances where the terminally ill person has little or no previous personal experience in religion, esoteric beliefs might become a first-time option.

Certainly, as previously indicated, dying people will often say and do almost anything to save their lives and often even their souls as well. On the night before her execution by hanging on July 7, 1865, for her role in a conspiracy to assassinate President Abraham Lincoln, Mary Surratt wept profusely while with two Catholic priests—whose prayers and statements about the Lord failed to calm her terrified heart and soul.

Life is a predicament which precedes death.
                                                            -Henry James

"Mrs. Surratt is innocent—she doesn't deserve to die with the rest of us," was the last statement by Lewis Powell, one of three men sentenced to hang along with the woman for their complicity in Lincoln's murder.

No amount of prayer and belief in the Lord could convince the fellow Christians within the U.S. government and Army to spare Surratt's life.

Cases of people condemned to die via execution or via natural causes including cancer continually signify that human life ends for us all, no matter what our beliefs.

Even so, a belief in traditional or non-traditional religious or spiritual beliefs often comforts both the dying and those they leave behind.

"He's with the Lord now, finally, thank God," becomes a typical comment from surviving relatives who refuse to accept the declaration by some scientists that "once it's over, it's over for good." The many dozens of religions or spiritual belief systems that have come, gone or remain hold little significance in the minds of scientific researchers.

I have no fear of death. More important, I don't fear life.
-Steven Seagal

Definitions of the afterlife and its meanings vary significantly among the various basic categories of religions—ranging from Christianity to Judaism and Islam.

For many sects of Buddhism, Hinduism, Theosophists, Jains, Sikhs, and other religions the afterlife is merely a temporary way station—a stopping place between the continual repitition of returning to life, ultimately ending in Nirvana.

Those who embrace most other standard religions aren't "as lucky," at least in the sense that their belief systems specify that we essentially have only one chance at eternal redemption via our actions in a single human life.

Thus, a dying person with numerous admitted failures in this life often feels a sense of loss and worry, thinking "will I become condemned for all eternity for my sins?"

Thankfully, at least in a spiritual or religious sense, many religions have given their members or parishioners a bit of wiggle room—a chance to redeem their souls.

Death in itself is nothing; but we fear to be we know not what, we know not where.
-John Dryden

For Catholics, redemption and a potential doorway to the Lord's Heavenly Kingdom swings wide open for dying sinners who sincerely and openly ask God for forgiveness of their sins.

Those who successfully ask for redemptions, in accordance with the specific rules or beliefs of their own particular sector, often open up the possibility of going to heaven.

Many times I've seen such belief systems serve as a motivation for dying people. To these individuals and their families such behavior makes perfect sense, particularly if they've been involved in an organized church.

And who could blame them?

It doesn't take a scientific public opinion poll to determine where dying people would want to go, either heaven or the repulsive opposite of that realm.

Abrahamic religions derived from the Middle East—Christian, Islam, Jewish and the Bahá'í Faith—all generally embrace as true the concepts of heaven and hell.

Since early childhood many of us were taught that heaven is a place for eternal salvation, an eternal dwelling site for the righteous. This is the complete opposite of hell, a place of eternal torment for the souls of people who were wicked in life such as Adolph Hitler.

James W. Forsythe, M.D., H.M.D.

In the first book of my Discworld series, published more than 26 years ago, I introduced Death as a character—there was nothing particularly new about this. Death has (been) featured in art and literature since medieval times, and for centuries we have had a fascination with the Grim Reaper.

-Terry Pratchett

Most "rules" set in stone by Abrahamic religions require that the one-way ticket to get into heaven is either good deeds performed during life or having faith while on Earth.

Needless to say, when visiting the hospital patient rooms or hospices of dying patients I have frequently encountered them and their families reading Bibles, reciting Holy Rosaries or engaging in a variety of other religious ceremonies.

Much of the time these are people who previously had given me no signal whatsoever that they were religious or God fearing in any way.

The sudden rush to God hails as an inalienable right within American society. As a devout Christian myself, I fully understand and empathize with these behaviors. Those embracing Islamic and Jewish traditions for the dying gain my additional respect.

Sometimes when I see people weeping in advance of their own death, I sense on occasion that this sometimes involves regrets for things done or undone in the past—along with regrets regarding whether they have fulfilled their own religion's specifications regarding God's wishes.

As the fly bangs against the window attempting freedom while the door stands open, so we bang against death ignoring heaven.

-Douglas Horton

In numerous cases while serving as chief of oncology, virtually every hospital where I have worked has featured a chapel designated as a quiet, personal place for worship.

About Death

For countless generations many cultures and societies have erected places of religious worship at locations where people are born and die.

Such traditions go as far back to the birth of Greek mythology, which initially embraced the concept that heroic people or relatives of gods might gain admission to an afterlife. Under the Greek belief system the definition of people qualified to enter this realm was expanded to include people who were good and kind while alive.

Whatever their particular beliefs, cultures and religions, for thousands of years most people have naturally had difficulty and fear when faced with the dying process.

Back then people had much more difficulty in avoiding issues of death than those who live today. Life expectancies during the Roman Empire were usually 35 to 40 years; many people never lived long enough to see their eventual grandchildren. Circumstances forced huge percentages of young children to participate in the burials of their young parents.

The spread and growth of belief systems that eventually evolved into many of today's mainstream religions provided at least some mental comfort. The vast majority of people as recently as a few hundred years ago were uneducated, depending on their churches for guidance on critical spiritual issues and almost anything that involved death.

In the last analysis, it is our conception of death which decides our answers to all the questions that life puts to us.

-Dag Hammarskjold

Specific belief systems regarding death and the afterlife gradually evolved or were modified in subsequent centuries.

For instance, contrary to popular belief the concept of "limbo" was not developed during Christ's era—but rather much later during the Middle Ages—a 1,000-year period from the Sixth

Century through the 15th Century.

Long after the crucifixion of Jesus Christ, theologians created the concept of limbo, designated as a place for the souls of innocent non-baptized people. Neither connected to heaven nor hell, limbo is defined as a place for the souls of various people, such as infants who never got baptized or adults who lived virtuous lives but never "embraced or lived the teachings of the Lord and Savior, Jesus Christ."

Such an otherworldly banishment in the afterlife may have motivated at least some people to join and participate in various Christian sects. Limbo was designated for good-hearted individuals who failed to take such action, partly because people outside of religion were deemed unqualified to commit personal sin—having never been baptized.

More than 500 years after the end of the Middle Ages, in the 21st Century the former Pope Benedict XVI, abolished the concept of limbo. This is just one of many examples of how religions have changed their rules or beliefs regarding death.

Sinful and forbidden pleasures are poisoned bread; they may satisfy appetite for the moment, but there is death in them at the end.
                                                            -Tyron Edwards

Besides heaven, hell and limbo, another afterworld location closely associated with the Catholic Church is purgatory. This supposedly is a stopping station, a place where the souls of certain dead people go for a period of time while ultimately en route to heaven.

People who have been non-sinful in a life that was filled with grace and friendship, but who remained imperfectly purified while alive deserve eternal life in heaven. But they first must be purified in purgatory if during life they failed to actively pursue the Word of the Lord. Without the fiery cleansing provided by purgatory, these souls lack the holiness necessary to gain admission into heaven.

Some scriptures refer to purgatory as having a cleansing fire although not permanent like hell's eternal flames. Some Christians refer to this way-station as having a "cleansing fire," while they avoid using the equally scary term "purgatory."

Once again the belief systems of particular religions or the various sects that such belief systems inspire retool much of society's rules and beliefs regarding the afterlife. Occasionally this is done to fulfill the personal whims and beliefs of church leaders at any specific point in time.

A key example of such changing rules occurred when John Wesley, a founder of Methodism, decided to embrace an "intermediate state" between death and Christianity's promised "resurrection of the dead." Unlike Catholics, many Methodists do not believe that prayer by living people will help the souls of people now ensconced in purgatory.

Poor Georgia O'Keeffe. Death didn't soften the opinions of the art world toward her paintings.
    -Jerry Saltz

The New Testament of the Bible tells us that Christ was able to rise up from the dead three days after his crucifixion. Christians celebrate his resurrection on Easter Sunday.

Since Christianity remains the most prevalent religious belief system in the United States, many dying people in our society look to Jesus' resurrection as a sign of hope.

Often beginning when they were mere toddlers many Christians have been taught that "Christ died for our sins." To the hearts of many dying people this concept brings hope for their own salvation, that they can indeed enter a positive afterlife—as long as they seek forgiveness for their sins and open up their souls to the way of the Lord.

James W. Forsythe, M.D., H.M.D.

Yet the specific beliefs regarding the afterlife often vary widely throughout the wide spectrum of Christianity. For instance, according to the Encyclopedia Britannica—just like limbo as mentioned earlier—the concept of purgatory was largely a result of the imagination of medieval Christians.

When becoming aware of these numerous conflicting and evolving beliefs, how should dying people and their families react when seeking guidance and help from their Christian churches?. What is a dying Christian in today's society expected to believe regarding such conflicting declarations regarding an afterlife?

To me, the answer seems obvious. Ultimately, only the terminally ill person and his family can decide for themselves. Rather than viewing this option as a "difficult situation," let us view the process as an opportunity to benefit from deep, abiding faith.

When I'm lying in my bed I think about life and I think about death, and neither one appeals to me.
-Steven Morrissey

The perceptions of a possible afterlife among most of today's dying people in the United States is vastly different from other cultures—particularly when compared to thousands of years ago during the Greek and Egyptian empires.

Historians and archeologists tell us that the Egyptians were among the first people in recorded history to develop a concept of the afterlife.

Within the ancient Egyptian culture people believed that upon death the soul breaks into parts—one the "ka" or body-double, and also into the personality referred to as "ba." Upon death, these sections would go to the Kingdom of the Dead.

Once in the afterlife the souls must pass a variety of tests in order to ultimately achieve the hoped-for goal of the ideal place within that realm. Entry required a sin-free heart, coupled with the ability to pass tests such as reciting details learned during life.

About Death

Early belief systems such as these were subsequently adopted by other cultures or societies, with specific requirements and definitions of the afterlife often hinged or fully devoted to the teachings of a particular religion's original spiritual leader.

Benjamin Franklin said there are only two things certain in life: death and taxes. But I'd like to add a third certainty: trash. And while some in this room might want to discuss reducing taxes, I want to talk about reducing trash.
-Ruth Ann Minner

Theologians say that the ancient Greeks played an integral role in generating a belief system that acknowledged the opposite of heaven—a hellish place originally called Hades. Actually, this was the name of a Greek God, who ruled the underworld.

Without any question whatsoever, people in the final stages of dying today want to stay as far away as possible during the afterlife from hell—which today's Christians believe is ruled by an evil entity known as the devil, Lucifer, the black angel or a fallen former devotee of God known by a variety of other names.

Biblical teachings such as these generate even more motivation for dying people to seek redemption for their sins. For them the choice becomes clear.

The downward option becomes unthinkable and even unmentionable. Under the Christian way of thinking and even within some Jewish teachings, hell remains an eternal place of damnation where the souls of sinful people are condemned to dwell forever.

These visions are so powerful even for non-believers who have never embraced Abrahamic beliefs that when in battle we tend to demonize our enemies.

There's nothing like pending death to rouse you from existential boredom.
-Roger Ebert

James W. Forsythe, M.D., H.M.D.

When imminently facing potential death on the battlefields of the world throughout history warriors have been taught to think of their adversaries as "the devil."

By adopting a "we-are-the-good-guys" mindset, soldiers from diverging armies are taught to avoid any fear of death because they're at battle against the Great Demon.

In a sense, as I've witnessed many times, a similar mindset has been carried over into modern culture in instances where a terminally ill person has cancer.

The mindset of the dying person and their relatives often evolves into an imaginary scene where the ill person becomes a warrior battling the disease—which is now being deemed a Wicked Demon.

Ultimately, almost everyone involved knows that—unless sent into a much-wanted state of remission—this "devil inside the body will eventually win out, resulting in its own death and that of its victim."

Yet like the soldiers at war on a battlefield, the dying person is said to have put up a "valiant and brave fight." This terminology usually gets passed onto a brief phrase or two in the person's obituary.

The general public's mindset, in indirect terms at least, tells us that the dead person has emerged as the actual winner—essentially gaining a one-way ticket to heaven simply for fighting the Big Feared Devil—cancer.

Particularly in today's highly competitive society, the general mindset dictates that people who fight their utmost against evil deserve a reward—in this case eternal salvation, a one-way ticket straight to heaven.

See, I have set before you this day life and good, death and evil...I have set before you life and death, blessing and curse, therefore choose life.

-Moses

About Death

Far from the Middle East where Abrahamic religions surfaced, separate belief systems in the Norway region also embraced their own concept of the afterlife.

People in the much colder north developed various beliefs based largely on poetic or Pose Edda literature generated in isolated regions including Iceland.

Yes, the yearning for living people to gain some sense of meaning and hope regarding the afterlife spread worldwide as various cultures and civilizations prospered.

Perhaps the most legendary of these Norse traditions and beliefs focused on Valhalla in Asgard, where the "chosen ones" go after death. Tradition dictated that half of warriors killed in battle would receive the honor of going to Valhalla in the afterlife.

The other half of warriors killed in battle would go to Fólkvangr, a great meadow known as Field of the Host, where they would join a beloved goddess, Freyja. A distinct figure in Norse mythology, people throughout that early culture associated her with death—plus war, gold, fertility, beauty, sexuality and love.

Some accounts of Freyja were first compiled in the 13th Century, long after the Roman, Greek, Egyptian and Abrahamic versions of the afterlife were created.

You have never seen death? Look in the mirror and you will see it like bees working in a glass hive.
                                                                    -Jean Cocteau

Anyone dying today might take comfort in knowing that these many belief systems have served people well throughout diverse cultures across several millennia.

Psychologists and other experts in the brain's complex functions generally believe that our thinking process can be used as a formidable tool.

Indeed, remember as previously stated, I've witnessed numerous occasions where a strong belief system significantly helps dying people, both mentally and spiritually. Aspects of some religions in a specific culture have been so strong that they become accepted in different regions.

One of the many examples of this involves early Jewish mystics who accepted reincarnation as a "real" God-given process, although this continual-life was first developed in the ancient culture of India vastly different from their own.

As indicated earlier, this contrasts with the Christian belief that holds we live only one earthly life.

Christians praise the words and promises of Jesus, who compared the Kingdom of Heaven with when fishermen throw a net into the sea to capture many kinds of fish. These men then sort though the entire catch, keeping the good and discarding the bad.

Believers insist that this is what will happen on the "Last Day," when God's loyal angels throw evil souls into the eternal damnation of hell—while sending righteous souls toward a light where they'll dwell in a heavenly kingdom with the Holy Father.

Science without conscience is the death of the soul.

-**Francois Rabelais**

Even Christians disagree on how the soul gets into heaven. Some believers claim that a ticket to entry can only be earned via appropriate behavior and worship in this lifetime. Others insist that the pearly gates open due to God's unmerited grace.

Numerous Christians such as Seventh-Day Adventists believe that upon the Second Coming of Christ, heaven will become possible to redeemed souls who are resurrected at that time.

Many other religions have vastly different versions of heaven and hell, plus unique ways to enter God's kingdom. The religions that all embrace vastly different beliefs about the Lord's Holy eternal place include Islam, Suni, Shia, Bahá'í Faith, Hinduism, Buddhism, Sikhism and others.

About Death

Mindful of these differences, some dying people choose to believe that all religions and spiritual belief systems are mere inventions of mankind. Others claim that assertions such as this are blasphemous and sacrilegious, since the "Word of the Lord" should be considered irrefutable.

On occasion I feel at least some sense of sorrow when witnessing a dying person who flat-out refuses to believe anything whatsoever.

Remember my previous declarations that a percentage of terminally ill people get locked in so much anger or sorrow that they refuse to consider any positive possibilities.

Life can't defeat a writer who is in love with writing, for life itself is a writer's lover until death.

-Edna Ferber

For dying people who have never attended church and lack religious education, there are no basic, universally accepted answers on where to seek answers regarding faith.

When and if a terminally ill person asks for my advice on this, I can tell them: "First, you need to move past any denial and anger that you might have at this point."

Then, breathe deeply and slowly for a period of time if your physical condition makes doing so possible. Gently calm your body and your mind, initially concentrating only on your breathing while fully relaxing all your muscles.

At the point where you enter deep mental and physical relaxation, start looking to your heart and soul for answers where your faith might lead your soul and mind.

Remember, I am not a spiritual counselor or a preacher, and would never strive to perform such functions. Only you can generate the best answers and beliefs for yourself, particularly at this phase of your life and at this point in time.

Based on what I've seen from past experience, important

answers can and will come to you—but only after such time as you can begin to truly love yourself and to appreciate what your own unique place has been within this universe.

We know the road to freedom has always been stalked by death.

-**Angela Davis**

Chapter 17
"Spooky" Belief Systems

The study and beliefs regarding death enter a unique realm when practitioners of parapsychology get involved. First developed in 1889 by Max Dossier, parapsychology entails a vast realm of what many people call "paranormal phenomenon."

Besides the concept of near-death experiences, these seemingly inexplicable beliefs delving into the afterlife include many differing or interrelated types of phenomenon. Some of the most widely known include clairvoyance, telepathy, psychokinesis, reincarnation and "seeing ghosts."

Practitioners and believers of parapsychology want to be perceived as serious and highly professional scientific-based people. Any declaration that these individuals are merely crackpots or "whacko" is considered offensive and politically incorrect, at least in much of today's world.

Nonetheless, the practice of or descriptions of parapsychologists is considered by some people as "abnormal" or controversial. Striving to ignore such criticisms, parapsychologists strive to steer away from such complaints while often investigating death-related matters.

Since the late 1800s intense study by these researchers has focused partly on whether the body truly has a soul and how living people communicate with the dead.

Man has but three events in his life: to be born, to live and to die. He is conscious of his birth, he suffers at his death and he forgets how to live.
                                                                -Jean de la Bruyere

James W. Forsythe, M.D., H.M.D.

Just 12 years after the formal creation of the parapsychology, in 1901 Massachusetts physician Duncan MacDougall conducted one of the first known scientific experiments in an attempt to determine whether living human bodies have souls.

Determined to get definitive, irrefutable scientific answers on this for the first time in history, MacDougall went to an old-age home where he weighed six patients while they were dying from tuberculosis. Notations made by the physician during this research mentioned that he had determined with relative ease when death was imminent.

Within a few hours of expected death, the doctor ordered that the patient's bed be placed on an industrial-size scale capable of measuring weights to the gram.

The subsequent findings of this physician emerged as intriguing to medical professionals, experts in theology, Christians and members of other religions.

In most of the six cases that MacDougall initially studied at the exact moment of death, the scale detected a loss in mass.

Does this mean that our bodies truly have souls, which leave our corpses at the moment of death?

If you make every game a life and death proposition, you're going to have problems. For one thing, you'll be dead a lot.

-Dean Smith

MacDougall used the measurable results in supporting or developing his hypothesis that as the soul leaves the body, so does a measurable amount of mass.

Highly controversial at the time but little-known by the USA's general population today, the doctor concluded that the average soul weighs 21 grams. That total was the average loss in mass as measured upon the death of the six test subjects.

Determined to intensify and to spread the scope of his research, MacDougall then measured sheep before and immediately after their deaths. These results showed that the animals briefly gained weight right after dying, additional mass that soon disappeared.

The physician then used the results involving the dead sheep in developing his additional hypothesis that a "portal" forms in the body upon death—from which the soul gets whisked away.

At this point MacDougall measured 15 dogs before and immediately after their deaths, failing to detect any discernable change in mass. Results from the canine experiments led him to theorize that the souls of people have weight and that dogs lack souls.

For three days after death, hair and fingernails continue to grow, but phone calls taper off.
                                                                                    -Johnny Carson

In 1907, six years after MacDougall's research began the "New York Times" broke the story as accounts of the experiments also were published in the "American Medicine" medical journal and the "Journal of the American Society for Physical Research."

Many scientists today consider the doctor's research as "false," citing the flawed methods of weighing the newly dead people and animals. In 2009, the Princeton University Press published results of a similar recent 21st Century study; the latest high-tech measuring devices failed to detect any measurable difference in weight upon death.

Despite these updated findings, many people throughout today's society still embrace apparent myth passed on through generations—still proclaiming that "the soul weighs 21 grams."

Nevertheless, hospital nurses and physicians in recent decades have occasionally told of strange or unexpected phenomenon immediately after a patient dies.

Some observers insist that they became startled upon briefly witnessing faint lights starting right after death or sometimes strange, inexplicable odors that soon disappeared.

James W. Forsythe, M.D., H.M.D.

Death comes in a flash, and that's the truth of it, the person's gone in less than 24 frames of film.

-Martin Scorsese

One of my friends in Reno swears that at the very moment his father died at home, a framed photograph of the newly deceased man fell off a wall at the home of a relative clear on the other side of town.

Dying people who hear such tales, particularly from people who swear that they're true, might tend to believe that, "There could be something there. Maybe the true inner me, my soul, will never die after all although my body will stop. I hope that's the case."

Even so, these terminally ill people also might want to know that some researchers in parapsychology including Susan Blackmore have concluded after more than 20 years of intense study that "there is no empirical evidence of an afterlife."

Such assertions are sharply disputed by others within this scientific field. David Fontana, a late British author, psychologist and academic, had insisted that evidence of an afterlife became so strong that everyone who closely studies the issue becomes convinced that our souls move to a new realm after death.

Fontana had stressed his opinion that any irrefutable, conclusive evidence "confirmed by scientists" that the afterlife exists would have merely become a chapter in a textbook. For him, the process of probing and continually researching the issue helps the mind develop.

There is no fundamental difference between the preparation for death and the practice of dying, and spiritual practice leading to enlightenment.

-Stanislov Grof

About Death

As this dispute between mainstream scientists and parapsychologists intensified in recent decades, some researchers in the paranormal have strived to scientifically search for our souls. At least one expert, mathematical physicist Frank J. Tripler, reportedly has argued that immortality can be proven by physics.

Yet according to at least one 1997 publication by Anchor Press, the late Austro-British professor Sir Karl Raimund Popper, widely regarded as among the greatest philosophers of science, proclaimed that Tripler's arguments should be discounted.

Popper reportedly argued that Popper's theory lacks any basis in science, largely because his claims of an existing afterlife could not be proven as "falsifiable or false."

Seeming to back up or fortify Tripler's theories, in 2008 an intensive care nurse in Great Britain, Penny Sartori, published a book about the near-death experiences of patients.

The nurse wrote that these people told her that they had floated above their own bodies. These individuals also giving her intricate and correct detail on medical procedures performed on them while clinically dead or unconscious.

Death consists, indeed, in a repeated process of unrobing, or unsheathing. The immortal part of man shakes off from itself, one after the other, its outer casings, and—as the snake from its skin, the butterfly from its chrysalis—emerges from one after another, passing into a higher state of consciousness.

-Annie Besant

Among their numerous realms of research, parapsychologists also study events that they label as "apparitional experiences."

Throughout human history people from numerous vastly diverse societies have reported seeing ghosts, apparitions or at least "visible spirits" of the dead.

For obvious reasons such assertions emerge as spooky,

otherworldly, or highly improbable at least in the minds of many people. Yet such claims fail to erase the fact that many people including some doctors and nurses insist that they have seen ghosts.

Several eminent scholars began attempting to scientifically research this controversial and highly disputed topic, beginning in 1882 when they formed the Society for Psychical Research. The organization became dedicated from its onset to the research of psychic and paranormal phenomenon.

Still existing today, based in London and conducting research worldwide, the society continues to press forward in a continual quest for definitive answers on these issues.

Deep down, no one really believes that they have a right to live. But this death sentence generally stays tucked away, hidden beneath the difficulty of living. If that difficulty is removed from time to time, death is suddenly there, unintelligibly.

-Jean Baudrillard

Before wondering to themselves whether "I'm going to become a ghost," today's terminally ill people need to realize that in the eyes of many skeptics the findings of the society and various parapsychologists remain inconclusive.

In originally creating its name, the Society adopted the term "psychical" in an attempt to differentiate itself from individuals or organizations labeled as psychic.

Reports of experiencing encounters with apparitions or seeing ghosts have continued worldwide since the Society was formed.

But at least judging from the literature that I have reviewed, parapsychologists and Society representatives have never scientifically proven that those supposed ghosts exist.

During my career including those many instances while with patients when they died, I have never encountered that I perceived a ghost or apparition.

About Death

Although lacking any solid personal opinion on this matter, I naturally become curious when hearing such stories. Some people might incorrectly assume that as a doctor with a scientific background I immediately designate such reports as bogus or unfounded.

As long as you don't make waves, ripples, life seems easy. But that's condemning yourself to impotence and death before you are dead.

-Jean Moreau

Chapter 18
Death-Defying Acts Abound

Throughout history people from many cultures have been so fascinated by the danger of death that they have been willing to see performers risk their lives.

Harry Houdini, a world-renowned stunt performer considered by some as perhaps history's greatest escape artist, often felt great pleasure in debunking the claims of spiritual mediums who had made bogus claims of communicating with the dead.

A native of Austria-Hungary born as "Eric Weisz" in Budapest in 1874, Houdini escaped almost certain death countless times during his illustrious career at entertainment venues across Europe and North America.

Muscular, determined and highly skilled at slight-of-hand techniques, his most famous escapes were from: handcuffs that a newspaper claimed were infallible; a sealed oversize milk can filled with water as the danger of possible drowning became imminent; and a famed Chinese Water Torture Cell in which he had been chained upside down.

Continually striving to generate new excitement, Houdini's many other successful acts during the first quarter of the 20th Century included being buried alive and slithering out of a nailed and roped packing crate that had been submerged in water.

About Death

Everything one does in life including love occurs in an express train racing toward death. To smoke opium is to get out of the train while it is still moving. It is too concern oneself with something other than life or death.

-Jean Cocteau

Long after a brief successful movie career, Houdini died October 31, 1926, in Detroit, Michigan, at age 52—the specifics of his death initially covered in a shroud of mystery. Various news reports claimed that the entertainer was killed by a bout of peritonitis, which had resulted from an appendicitis attack.

Some journalists subsequently quoted witnesses who claimed that they had seen J. Gordon Whitehead, a McGill University student, suddenly and unexpectedly slugging the entertainer's abdomen numerous times while in a theater dressing room.

As reported by the news media, at least two witnesses independently gave similar accounts, insisting that Whitehead had essentially asked Houdini if it were true that punches to the stomach would fail to hurt him.

The reporters quoted Sam Smilovitz and Jacques Price—named in some accounts as Sam Smiley and Jack Price—as saying they heard Houdini give Whitehead permission to slug him. Without hesitation the student summarily walloped his own fists in rapid-fire succession below the entertainer's beltline.

The famed escape artist soon asked the student to stop, telling the young man that he had not had time to prepare for receiving the blows—having not expected Whitehead to hit with such sudden ferocity.

The famed writer, Author Canon Doyle, creator of the fictional, iconic Sherlock Holmes detective character, wrote in 1930 five years after Houdini's death that a broken ankle that Houdini had suffered several days before the incident had prevented him from standing up straight enough to brace his body from the blows.

James W. Forsythe, M.D., H.M.D.

Whenever I watch TV and see all those poor starving kids all over the world, I can't help but cry. I mean I'd love to be skinny like that, but not with all those flies and death and stuff.

-Mariah Carey

That evening after being punched Houdini performed his act while suffering extensive pain caused by the incident. Perhaps pride had prevented the entertainer from seeking medical help during the next few days as his pain intensified.

By the time Houdini finally visited a physician the entertainer's temperature had jumped above 102 degrees. A doctor diagnoses appendicitis and advised immediate surgery. Yet reporters later chronicled the fact that Houdini refused to undergo the potentially life-saving operation, choosing instead to "go on with the show."

The decision proved fatal, as the performance became the entertainer's last. By this point his fever had spiked to 104 degrees. Some accounts claim that Houdini passed out during his show, only to be revived before vowing to complete his performance.

"I'm tired of fighting," Houdini was quoted as saying shortly before his death, as quoted in a 2006 book by William Kalush and Larry Sloman, published by Simon & Schuster, "The Secret Life of Houdini: The Making of America's First Superhero."

Today, for terminally ill people and for those us who are afraid of dying, the true-life story of Houdini's demise should serve as an essential lesson—that even the world's greatest, most highly acclaimed escape artist cannot escape eventual death.

You know Americans are obsessed with life and death and rebirth, that's the American Cycle. You know, awakening, tragic, horrible death and then Phoenix rising from the ashes. That's the American story, again and again.

-Billy Corgan

About Death

Many people watching movies and live performances seemingly pay little or no attention to the fact that people are literally risking their life for someone's viewing pleasure.

This factor signifies just one of the many amazing or intriguing things about death. People rarely want to talk about the subject or to think of their own eventual demise. Yet they're often innately fascinated when watching such performances.

Those putting their lives on the line range from trapeze artists and lion tamers to motorcyclists and racecar drivers. They're often called "daredevils," "stuntmen" or "stunt performers."

Audiences reacted in a display of shock, tears and screams upon seeing motorcyclist Evel Knievel's body get pulverized in a stunt mishap at Caesars Palace in Las Vegas on New Year's Eve in 1967.

The crowd wailed in tears of grief when tightrope walker Karl Wallenda fell to his death at age 73 in San Juan, Puerto Rico, when attempting to walk along a wire between two hotels. His great-grandson, Nik Wallenda, continues to perform today—successfully walking a high-wires across the Grand Canyon, and also above Niagara Falls.

In sleep we lie all naked and alone, in sleep we are united at the heart of night and darkness, and we are strange and beautiful asleep; for we are dying the darkness and we know no death.

-Thomas Wolfe

One of the most shocking and surprising daredevil accidents resulted in critical injuries suffered by entertainer Roy Horn—from the famed, internationally acclaimed duo Siegfried & Roy; he had often appeared with white lions and white tigers.

During a show at the Mirage in Las Vegas on October 3, 2003, a 7-year-old male tiger, Montecore, bit Horn's neck.

The entertainer suffered severe blood loss as stage crews separated Horn from the tiger before paramedics rushed the man in critical condition to Nevada's only Level 1 trauma facility, University Medical Center.

Horn underwent several years of continuous physical rehabilitation therapy. His entertainment partner, Siegfried Fischbacher, later said during a TV show appearance that the tiger had acted as such an animal would in the wild, attempting to drag Horn as if the man were a cub after the entertainer fell onto the stage during the show.

Once again, the Siegfried & Roy tragedy marked just one of the many daredevil stunts gone awry. Yet many of us within the general public still eagerly buy expensive tickets to see such "death-defying shows."

Perhaps at least for some of us this stems partly from an apparent deep inner "blood-thirstiness." As the mainstream media continually chronicles the advice of politicians and charities urging people to show compassion for one another, our hearts sometimes seem undeniably cold when given the opportunity to watch others face potential death.

Death is inevitable, but life—that's a tricky bit where things happen.

-Simon Travaglia

Chapter 19

Humanity's Quest for Massive Death

Human sacrifice, the intentional killing of other people for entertainment, pleasure or religious reasons, has occurred on every continent except Antarctica throughout the course of human history.

Outlawed today on a worldwide scale, the once-accepted process of intentionally killing people in public places has occurred in almost every major country that eventually became "civilized."

One of the most infamous venues for killing people as a form of blatant public entertainment occurred at the Colosseum in Rome—which still stands in ruins as a significant tourist attraction.

Heralded as the largest amphitheater during the Roman Empire, built nearly 2000 years ago and about 75 years after Christ's death, the facility hosted up to up 80,000 people who cheered while watching condemned pre-determined victims die horrific bloody deaths.

Today, people suffering from painful terminal illnesses while in hospitals, hospices or at home do not have to worry about being stomped by elephants, eaten alive by lions or impaled by a gladiator's sharp weapons.

I was perfectly content before I was born, and I think of death as the same state. What I am grateful for is the gift of intelligence, and for life, love, wonder and laughter. You can't say it wasn't interesting. My lifetime's memories are what I have brought home from the trip.
                                                            -Roger Ebert

James W. Forsythe, M.D., H.M.D.

The values, laws and morals of today's society, particularly within the United States, requires that people officially refrain from even entertaining the idea of such blatant cruelty.

Yet as disturbing as this fact might seem, it's true: some religions and politicians throughout history have required human sacrifices as an accepted part of culture or of religious doctrine.

A huge portion of history's many instances of human sacrifice have involved religious ritual killings. These often involved methodically and intentionally murdering one or more people simultaneously as a sacrifice to perceived gods or creators.

Many adults today worry about their own impending deaths from diseases such as cancer. Children and entire families from the past often had much different fears, primarily dying via stones or weapons inflicted upon them during human sacrifice.

Some highly demented and warped rules even required the massive, simultaneous killings of a monarch's slaves. The killers performed these heinous acts under the misguided belief that the slain would be able to serve their late master in the afterlife.

People always say that pregnant women have a glow. And I say it's because you're sweating to death.
-Jessica Simpson

Headhunters or cannibals from some societies preferred to slaughter people from other tribes or nations as a sacrifice to their gods.

By the Iron Age from the late 1700s to the mid-1800s, the massive worldwide traditions of human sacrifice finally began to wane—at least on a widespread, generally accepted international scale. But today's sociologists and archeologists say ritual killings still leave a soiled mark on many of today's cultures.

Such customs are extremely rare today. In India, for instance, people in the Sati funeral tradition, typically threw widows onto the funeral pyres of their dead husbands—intentionally immolating the women.

About Death

Some of these widows intentionally jumped into the fires. Accurate, reliable historical records on these sacrifices remain scarce. Many historians believe the tradition began thousands of years ago, when mourners revered the dead women as objects of reverence and worship—sometimes individually referred to as the "good wife."

Upon learning of traditions such as this, many people in today's society would become understandably perplexed. Overall today's society, particularly in the Western culture, is said to value human life above almost everything else—except in matters of abortion and condemning convicted killers in an eye-for-an-eye process.

As long ago as 300 years before Christ, witnesses reported having seen the two wives of the same man fight each other for the right to throw themselves on his funeral pyre. Greek people became so mystified upon learning of such intentional sacrifices that they theorized that those traditions in India had been imposed to discourage young wives from intentionally poisoning their much older husbands.

The sunlight ranges over the universe, and at incarnation we step out of it into the twilight of the body, and see but dimly during the period of our incarceration; at death we step out of the prison again into the sunlight, and are nearer to the reality.

-Annie Besant

A less traditional, less frequent suicide method in ancient northern India did not involve only wives. Instead, anyone from both genders who knew the deceased was permitted to kill themselves at a loved one's funeral—often using poisons or weapons to end their lives rather than immolation.

The deceased person's relatives, friends, followers and friends were permitted to slaughter themselves—essentially "joining in on the death party."

James W. Forsythe, M.D., H.M.D.

During the 1500s, Muslim Mughals that invaded India refrained from stopping many of that region's long-term customs—except sati. A Mughal emperor went so far as to ban the custom, but Hindus resisted the new regulations because they liked their custom.

Today the idea of watching women burn themselves to death and to encourage the custom seems repulsive. Yet the people of long ago in India and many other cultures cherished their ability to slaughter other individuals or to watch them die.

Many people today who insist that most humans are "ignorant, poorly educated pigs who lack moral values" need look no further than such cultures of the relatively recent past. Some observers might even argue that the hearts and souls of many people today still remain as cold and as impersonal as ever, insensitive to the emotional and physical pains of others.

The Greeks said grandly in their tragic phrase, "let no one be called happy 'till his death;" to which I would add, "Let no one, 'till his death, be called unhappy."

　　　　　　　　　　　　　　　　-Elizabeth Barrett Browning

No reliable statistics seem to exist today on the total estimated number of women who intentionally burned themselves to death in sati rituals. Yet the process continued for more than 300 years in various regions of India following the Muslin Mughal conquests—leading to the assumption that perhaps many hundreds of thousands of widows over time chose to immolate themselves above their husband's burning bodies.

These are just limited examples of human sacrifices that occurred on a worldwide scale over thousands of years. Perhaps millions of people collectively over time died painfully in this way in many cultures—either willingly or unwillingly.

A careful review of human sacrifice traditions points to religion and the beliefs in gods as the biggest culprit.

About Death

People allowed themselves to believe evil values that devalued human life, while placing much greater value on false gods such as the sun, golden statues or mystical fictitious entities that had merely been created in the warped minds of mere mortals.

Those of us reviewing these historical tragedies today are left to condemn the heartlessness of mankind. Ignorant people invariably feel a need to be "told what to do, and told how to think."

Rather than growing up permitted to have independent minds of their own, people were taught senseless, useless dogma beginning in early childhood. This creepy process often led to their own destruction or to a steady evolution into becoming killers as young adults.

At the solemn moment of death every man even when death is sudden, sees the whole of his past life marshaled before him, in its minutest details. For one short instant the personal becomes one with the individual and all-knowing ego. But this instant is enough to show to him the whole chain of causes which have been at work during his life.

-Annie Besant

The sati tradition in various regions of India finally began to subside in the 1800s when Sahajanand Swami, at the time leader of the increasingly dominant Swaminarayan sect, argued that no person has a right to take his or her own life—a gift that only God has a right to take or to give.

During the previous four millennia human sacrifice victims from various cultures apparently were given a choice of how they would die.

Archaeologists have concluded that until 2,800 years before Christ servants and high officials of dead kings were allowed to poison themselves. Similar suicide-by-poison options in Mesopotamia were given to guards, grooms, handmaidens and magicians of dead kings.

James W. Forsythe, M.D., H.M.D.

The Bible even mentions human sacrifice when the Lord tests Abraham by telling him to kill his son Isaac on Mount Moriah as an offering to God. Abraham refrains from protesting, and thankfully an Angel stops this man in time by providing a ram for the ritual, thereby preventing the murder of Isaac.

Countless other children in other countries weren't as lucky. Child sacrifice became common in the ancient cultures of Phoenicians and Carthaginians, according to old Greek and Roman sources.

I think about death a lot, like I think we all do. I don't think of suicide as an option, but as fun. It's an interesting idea that you can control how you go. It's this thing that's looming, and you can control it.

-Ryan Gosling

The value of human life seemed non-existent through much of Europe thousands of years before organized large civilizations emerged there. Archaeologists say that between 3,000 years and 2,000 years before Christ, people in the Yumna culture in what now is the Russian-Ukranian region slaughtered infants in rituals for their gods.

The ancient Hebrew Bible says the infants were cooked alive in a "roasting place" called a tophet; on orders from their religious leaders, many people willingly and eagerly cooked the babies alive to honor their gods, Baal and Moloch. The adults worshipped statues crafted to represent these deities.

According to various published reports, some archeologists including Jonathan N. Tubb have concluded that adults who willingly killed their babies were Canaanites who had settled farming villages as recently as 1,200 years before Christ.

The wretched capability and eagerness of people to slaughter their loved ones and neighbors occurred 4,000 years before Christ near Perevalsk in the Ukraine.

About Death

The relentless yearning to see blood flow later spread to the cultures of ancient Rome and Greece. Historical texts indicate that ancient Athenians participated in human sacrifices at the world-famous Acropolis of Athens, which still stands.

Human sacrifices became so popular that tales of such events spread into Greek mythology. The practice apparently was much less frequent in Rome before Christ, where people threw straw figures substituting for elderly men into the Tiber River.

One of the greatest gifts we can give people is the hope that their death is nothing to fear—you know, not that it has no fear in it, but the promise of scripture is that God will lead us through the valley of the shadow of death.
-Max Lucado

According to the writings of Roman Empire Emperor Julius Caesar, the Celts of central Europe—called "druids" or Gaul people—eagerly generated funeral pyres for the corpses of deceased high-ranking dead people; in the process, the druids supposedly burned the dead person's servants alive in the conflagration.

Caesar claimed that the Gaul people also forced streams of living people to go into large wicker figures imaged to look like a person, before the entire mass was set ablaze.

Other ancient writings claimed that the Gaul people had different methods of human sacrifice, each designed to honor a specific God.

Often after victories against Roman armies, the Gauls often supposedly drowned some captives to honor the god Toutatis.

Other captors honoring the god Taranis set their victims afire. With equal ferocity Gauls honoring the god Esus hanged their victims.

Some current archeologists dispute such claims of ancient Romans involving the Celts. Perhaps Roman rulers used bogus information for propaganda intended to portray their enemies as barbaric.

Death is a delightful hiding place for weary men.

-Herodotus

Theories of human sacrifices in early German society remain a matter of dispute. Prior to the Viking Age during the first and second centuries after Christ, the Roman senator Tacitus claimed that the Goths sacrificed prisoners of war before hanging the victims severed limbs from trees.

At least according to the writings of an ancient Arab traveler, Ahmad ibn Fadlan, who kept a historic journal of his journey from Baghdad to Volga Bulgaria, Norse warriors were sometimes buried with sacrificed enslaved women—due to a belief that the ladies would become their wives in Valhalla.

Imagery of the intense brutality becomes possible when learning of Fadlan's report that prior to the funeral of Scandinavian chieftains some enslaved women volunteered to die with a Norseman. Ten days of festivities followed these bizarre declarations, culminating when a designated old woman stabbed the volunteering lady to death.

People celebrating at the funeral then burned the dead lady's body along with the corpse of a sacrificed Norseman, the conflagration engulfing a boat containing the sacrificed woman and the deceased chieftain's body.

Some archaeologists reportedly have found evidence that this claim was true. Additional research indicates that the original ruler of the Vikings in Normandy, Rollo, allowed his people to appease the gods by participating in human sacrifices.

About Death

Your body must become familiar with its death—in all its possible forms and degrees—as a self-evident, imminent, and emotionally neutral step on the way towards the goal you have found worthy of your life.

-Dag Hammarskjold

    Systematic and continual human sacrifices also became common in the early years of the Slavic and Chinese cultures, archaeologists say. Besides occasionally burying slaves alive along with their owners who had died naturally, the ancient Chinese also are said to have drowned young men and young women as sacrifices to the gods of various rivers.

    Researchers indicate that these practices were prevalent during the Zhou and Shang dynasties between 200 and 2,000 years before Christ.

    Outraged by what had been done to their fellow countrymen, historians say, common people from that region worked together to write the poem "Yellow Bird."

    The famous phrases condemning these barbaric practices was done after the ruler Duke Wu had ordered 66 of his slaves killed upon his death 678 years before Christ. Eighteen years later, in 621 B.C., the ruler Duke Mu ordered that 177 of his slaves be slaughtered after he died.

    The rulers had ordered these mass killings, believing that the dead souls of the servants would provide companionship in the afterlife. Yet the "Yellow Bird" poem apparently failed to convince the wretched, self-centered rulers to end their barbaric custom.

    According to a 2012 article in the "New York Times," archaeologists have excavated the remains of 186 victims who had been buried along with Duke Jing of Qin. His reign ended upon his death in 537 B.C., nearly a century after the other sacrifices had inspired "Yellow Bird."

James W. Forsythe, M.D., H.M.D.

As a kid, all I thought about was death. But you can't tell your parents that.
-Maurice Sendak

Archaeologists have discovered additional instances of human sacrifices in Tibet, from the ancient Native Hawaiian culture, and in Pre-Colombian cultures in the Americas. Some of the most notorious human sacrifices occurred continuously over periods spanning many hundreds of years in Central America and North America.

Ruthless beliefs in the early Mayan culture in Central Mexico motivated people to throw their victims into huge limestone sinkholes, believed by them to be gateways to the underworld. Modern researchers there have found the remains of numerous victims, more than half of them under age 20.

The Aztec people of Mexico were even more bloodthirsty in their human sacrifices. By some estimates more than 80,000 prisoners were slain in these barbaric Aztec rituals, their hearts ripped out of their bodies while they were alive.

These rituals, in which tens of thousands of people were sacrificed in individual ceremonies, occurred a mere 500 years ago in the early 1500s. The senseless carnage finally ended during the height of that period upon the invasion of Christian Europeans.

At least one researcher, Michael Harner, estimated in a 1997 article that a whopping 250,000 people were sacrificed in Central Mexico during the early 1500s.

I was fascinated about my own death, I started thinking what my funeral would be like and what music would be played, I was at that level of insanity.
-Billy Corgan

Additional research by archaeologists across North American indicates that human sacrifices also became commonplace across a region that later became the United States.

About Death

Researchers have found the remains of many Native Americans, slain en masse hundreds of years ago in what is now Mississippi and Missouri.

Archaeologists believe that like many sacrifices in China, the mass slaughter of many hundreds of Native Americans occurred immediately after the natural deaths of their rulers. Some of these North American sacrificial killings reportedly occurred just 300 years ago.

Beside the body of the Natchez ruler Tattooed Serpant, who died in 1725, researchers have found the remains of numerous people who choose to die with him. These included a war clubs craftsman, his nurse, head servant, a doctor and a warrior.

South American cultures, particularly among the Incas, hundreds and thousands of years ago became equally morbid.

In the Moche Cultural region of Northern Peru, scientists have unearthed the remains of at least 40 male adolescents sacrificed between 200 and 800 years after Christ. These children were slain en masse after being defeated in ceremonial battles.

I don't think kids have a problem with death. It's us older ones who are nearer to it, that start being frightened.

-Helena Bonham Carter

Once again the Incans were among cultures worldwide that independently adopted a warped ideology dictating that servants of rulers be sacrificed for their masters' funerals.

Additionally bizarre human sacrifices occurred as recently as throughout western Africa, particularly after the death of a king or queen.

According to documentation from the time, hundreds or even thousands of slaves were sacrificed at single events.

"In one of these ceremonies in 1727, as many as many as 4,000 were reported killed," in Dahomey, a former African kingdom in what is now the Republic of Benin, wrote Rudolph

Rummel, a professor emeritus of political science at the University of Hawaii. Rummel also said that during that era in Dahomey authorities dictated an annual custom that mandated the sacrifice of at least 500 slaves every year.

Throughout nearly the first 1,800 years after Christ and for thousands of years prior, tribes across Asia and Africa engaged in cannibalism. Tribes tracked and murdered people, in part targeting their victims as a sacrifice to various gods.

People don't think that celebrities have to worry about things like sickness, and death, and rent. It's like you've traveled to this Land of Celebrity, this other country. They want you to tell about what you saw.
-David Duchovney

Disturbingly, many religions that remain dominant worldwide today featured early writings or scriptures that described human sacrifices in morbid detail.

The story previously mentioned regarding Abraham and his son Isaac, spared by an angel, is just one example.

Historians of Judaism have disagreed whether Jepthah mentioned in Hebrew biblical text carried out his vow to God to kill the first thing that came out of his door. Some accounts indicate Jepthah ordered his daughter to never marry, while others indicate that he burned his daughter alive

The concept of such senseless killings is so deep that—although some theologians disagree—numerous analysts have equated the crucifixion of Jesus Christ as a human sacrifice.

Elsewhere, throughout much of the history of Hinduism in India various spiritual leaders have embraced and endorsed human sacrifice—which they call "ahimas."

Disease, insanity and death were the angels that attended my cradle, and since then have followed me throughout my life.
-Edvard Munch

About Death

Allegations of human sacrifice continue today, with some protestors claiming that countries such as the United States send soldiers to get slaughtered—largely in the name of the "almighty dollar," derived from resources such as oil.

Proponents and opponents of the U.S. wars in Iraq and Afghanistan in the early 21st Century sharply disagree with each other on this factor.

A review of wars throughout history in many nations indicates there can be little doubt that the leaders of countries sacrifice the lives of their young adults—primarily men. The U.S. war in Vietnam and various military skirmishes involving Great Britain in recent decades have drawn complaints of soldiers sacrificed for economic reasons.

Some sociologists contend that the value of human life is often given little or no value by national leaders concerned primarily with protecting their political interests.

During the past century despots, warlords and dictators have ordered the indiscriminate slaughter of their own people in nations around the world.

Some of the most horrific have included Stalin of Russia, Hitler from Germany, Idi Amin of Uganda, and Pol Pot from Cambodia. Collectively these evil despots orchestrated, managed, ordered or condoned the slaughter and eradication of many millions of people.

Seasonal changes, as it were, take place in history, when there is practically an almost universal death, a falling of the foliage of the tree of life. Such were the intervals between the ancient and the mediaeval and the modern.

-George Edward Woodberry

Chapter 20

Death by Execution

Through these epic periods spanning thousands of years, mankind developed a wide variety of execution methods as punishment for real or supposed crimes.

Some countries once considered barbaric now ban executions, while some nations including the United States still sanction executions on a state-by-state basis.

Beginning in ancient times some of the most popular execution methods have included being stomped by elephants, getting ripped apart by a team of horses and planned attacks by scorpions, snakes and spiders.

Numerous societies have required that the condemned die as slowly and as painfully as possible, while other cultures strive to achieve instantaneous death.

In the Middle East and Persia some monarchs ordered soldiers to stomp horses above criminals, while the Mongols thousands of years ago preferred to snap the backs of victims partly in order to avoid spilling blood on the ground.

Our birth is nothing but our death begun, as tapers waste the moment they take fire.

-Edward Young

Determined to give the killings of perceived entertainment value, at least according to archeologists and historical texts, some condemned people were blown out of cannons.

About Death

Spectators in a variety of cultures got just as much delight when seeing the condemned get boiled to death, or when the condemned person's body was mangled in breaking wheels designed to slowly and meticulously snap bones.

Some of the loudest cheers of delight occurred when doomed people were slowly buried alive. During the Roman Empire such burials of living people were considered an ideal way to dispose of former vestal virgins who had broken their vows of chastity.

Although not perceived as quite as entertaining for viewers, drowning sometimes became popular as punishment for many types of criminal offenses. Due to intense public demand, some were drowned slowly—allowed to resurface for air every 20 seconds to 30 seconds for a lengthy period of time, until finally submerged until death.

Throughout Great Britain monarchs often preferred to have the condemned burned alive at the stake, usually in public places where the general public could cheer as the condemned screamed.

Often ordered to kill for religious reasons, executioners skilled at burning people alive often slowly cooked the victim's toes, feet, and lower legs. Well-honed at their cookery, the killers strived to create as much anguish as possible until the flames finally and gracefully engulfed the person and completed the deed.

Courage is the art of being the only one who knows you're scared to death.

-**Earl Wilson**

The cherished tradition of burning people alive was adopted in the new North American colonies in the 1500s. Although hanging often became a preferred method, people convicted of witchcraft were often burned alive in Europe and the Americas.

In Great Britain, particularly during the reigns of such monarchs as King Henry VIII and Queen Elizabeth I, the

James W. Forsythe, M.D., H.M.D.

condemned occasionally were hung by the neck for brief periods—finally taken from the noose still conscious. Then, the executioners would extract some of the person's intestines—careful to leave vital nerves in tact. The extracted organs were summarily cooked in a skillet, generating screams of pain.

This was often called "hanged, drawn and quartered." From the removal of intestines and perhaps other organs, the individual was chopped into four distinct parts that were subsequently sent to various regions for display as examples of what happens to those guilty of treason.

Perhaps just as cruelly, torture racks were sometimes designed to slowly pull the person's joints and internal organs apart—sometimes as the poor condemned person was being cooked as slowly as possible at a simmer.

Humanity's persistent inhumanity to man proved just as horrific a few thousand years ago when rulers occasionally stuffed the condemned into a hollow brazen bull with a door on the side—often called a "bronze bull" or a "Sicilian bull." The person was then slowly roasted to death as executioners subjected the container to intense heat.

The bull's devilish creators designed the head with compartments that made the person's screams sound like those of such an animal. Adding to the demented pleasures of delighted spectators, the contraption also was designed to emit unique aromas as the various roasting stages commenced.

According to legend, Phalaris, a former ruler who had first approved the designing and construction of the device was eventually executed in the contraption when his kingdom was overthrown.

Life isn't fair. It's just fairer than death, that's all.
                                                            -William Goldman

About Death

Some historians have claimed that early Romans used brazen bulls to slaughter Jews. Some Christians believe that Emperor Hadrian ordered the execution of Saint Eustace, simultaneously with his wife and children in a bronze bull or bronze ox in the second century after Christ.

Historical texts indicated that the tradition of using bronze bulls for executions lasted until nearly 500 years after Christ, when King Alaric II ordered the killing of a Roman usurper, Burdunellus.

Throughout that 1,000-year span elaborate torture chambers were sometimes used to extract information from people—with execution the ultimate objective.

Jesus Christ was among countless victims who suffered a torturous crucifixion death, in which the condemned were roped or nailed to trees, vertical poles or crosses. These condemned usually died from exposure to the elements, their wounds or starvation.

The methods of crushing people to death in various cultures in diverging eras included being smashed to death by boulders or elephants. When some spectators demanded that people being crushed die slowly and painfully, the executions would gradually and methodically place increasingly heavier objects onto the person's chest.

Some despotic or demented societies including the early Kingdom of Great Britain even demanded that the criminal suspect strive to verbally enter his plea of guilt or innocence at the point when the excessive weight makes breathing and speaking extremely difficult or impossible.

Witnesses reported in text accounts that such "pressing to death" sometimes took several days to complete, due to the extremely slow and methodical manner of adding weights after the condemned person's limbs were tied into different directions.

James W. Forsythe, M.D., H.M.D.

I was brought up by very witty people who were dealing with quite difficult things: disease and death...I was brought up by people who tended to giggle at funerals.

~ Emma Thompson

Beheading became a popular quick execution method in numerous cultures, particularly during the height of the French Revolution in the late 1700s.

Some cultures enjoyed disemboweling the condemned, literally taking their intestines out. Under normal circumstances people who are carved apart this way die within hours. For the viewing pleasure of ecstatic crowds after disemboweling a victim the executioner often pulled out the heart or severed the head.

According to witness accounts, the North Vietnamese sometimes disemboweled South Vietnamese peasants as a form of psychological intimidation toward their surviving relatives and neighbors.

One of the most popular execution methods in the United States became electrocution, particularly in numerous Southern states during the early and mid-20th Century. Upon the start of electric currents, the condemned's vital organs are fatally damaged. Death often occurs when electric currents over-stimulate the heart.

Although electrocution is no longer used frequently in the USA, this method remains an option for the condemned in several states. The vast majority of these prisoners instead choose death via lethal injection, which some scientists claim is relatively painless when correctly administered.

Many states eventually banned execution via electrocution, swayed by the argument that such deaths are cruel and unusual as prohibited by the U.S. constitution. Interestingly, this method had first been adopted by many states after 1881 when the state of New York deemed electricity as a humane and logical replacement to hanging.

About Death

We have a limit, a very discouraging, humiliating limit: death.

                                                          –Umberto Eco

Some societies have preferred to drop the condemned to their deaths, plummeting to the ground for great heights. Young healthy adults in pre-Roman Sardinia sometimes executed elderly people who were unable to care for themselves, throwing the condemned off cliffs after forcing the person to ingest intoxicating sardonic herbs.

A steep cliff called the Tarpeian Rock was sometimes chosen as the execution site for traitors and murderers during the Roman Republic, overlooking the Forum in ancient Rome. To some observers this execution carried a stigma of shame, a fate worse than death—condemned to die in this way rather than the standard form of strangulation.

Suetonius, a Roman historian who observed and documented historical events during the Roman Empire including the reign of Julius Caesar, watched as people convicted of sexual perversions and cruelty were thrown off a cliff into the sea.

Immediately following well-planned and meticulous torture sessions, these executions were often witnessed by the Emperor Tiberius, who had ordered the killings; he reigned from 14 years to 37 years after Christ. Any person "lucky" enough to survive the fall would summarily have his bones broken by people who waited at the bottom of the cliff.

Execution via dropping reportedly has occurred as recently as 2008, when news reports indicated that two men convicted of rape were thrown off a cliff or dropped from a tremendous height. Elsewhere, some people reportedly have made unverified claims that during the reign of Augusto Pinochet in Chile from 1974 to 1990 some condemned people were dropped to their deaths from helicopters.

James W. Forsythe, M.D., H.M.D.

Sleep is lovely, death is better still, not to have been born is of course the miracle.

-Heinrich Heine

A far more torturous and particularly cruel execution method used in diverse cultures involved "flaying," a term for skinning animals and people alive.

The Aztecs in Mexico sometimes flayed people during human sacrifice, and in some Persian or Middle East countries such as Iraq. The actual flaying process sometimes occurred after the victim had already died, but sometimes the skin-removal process was carried out while the person was still alive.

Strange religious beliefs sometimes dictated flaying; the dead person's skin was often wanted for supposed magical purposes or for use as a "deterrence" to discourage living people from contemplating or carrying out similar crimes.

When flaying was inflicted upon a live person the process was a chosen method for torture. Traitors often suffered this fate in medieval Europe. Crowds often cheered as the skin was cut and flayed from the body as slowly and methodically as possible.

This treacherous cruelty, deemed today as unthinkable or seemingly unimaginable, became a popular method of exterminating traitors in France during the 1700s.

Extremely graphic and repulsive descriptions of these executions were recounted in the 1975 book "Discipline and Punish," by the late French author, historian, literary critic and social theorist Michel Foucault.

Historians have insisted that at least three Chinese emperors that reigned several hundred years before Christ had summarily ordered skin removed for the faces of people who committed various crimes.

If historic documentation is correct, one of the cruelest by far was the Chinese Hongwu Emperor, who reigned for a 30-year period nearly 1,400 years after Christ. According to a 2001 report by Chinese Friendship Publishing Company, he ordered the flaying of a whopping 5,000 women, plus similar killings of rebels, corrupt officials and servants.

I hate death; it takes people away from you. You're left feeling rudderless.
-John Lydon

The many notorious documented flaying executions in the Western World have included: the skinning of Saint Bartholomew in Armenia in the first century after Christ; Pierre Basile, skinned alive in 1199 for the slaying of King Richard I of England; and two brothers who had become lovers of a daughter of King Philip IV of France were slowly skinned alive before being castrated and beheaded.

One of the most dumbfounding instances of execution was 1589 flaying of a Rhineland or West German woman, as punishment for supposedly "submitting" to incest or rape inflicted by her father, Peter Stumpp.

A wealthy farmer, suspected cannibal and serial killer, this man's crimes became so notorious that he earned the nickname "Werewolf of Bedburg." During torture on a rack he confessed to practicing "black magic," eventually resulting in what some historians have labeled perhaps one of the most notorious "werewolf trials" in history.

Simultaneously executed along with his daughter and his mistress, Peter Stumpp was first slowly flayed on ten separate places of his body. The executioners then placed him on a torture wheel, before torturing him further with red-hot pincers. Then, to the delight of the crowd, the executioners meticulously pulled all the skin from his arms and legs, slowly and delicately enough so that he would remain alive.

To prevent Stumpp from returning from his grave, the executioners then used axe handles to pulverize his legs. The man was then beheaded before the severed head and corpse were summarily burned. Just prior to killing Stubbs, the executioners flayed and raped his daughter and mistress. Adding to the drama, apparently drawing tremendous cheers from the blood-thirsty crowd, the women were then burned alive in the same fire that engulfed Stubbs' corpse.

Some critics have contended that the accusations, trial and execution of Stubbs actually had been politically motivated, because he had converted to Protestantism. Guilty or not, Stubbs became so notorious that his name was even mentioned in "The Exorcist," a 1971 supernatural suspense novel by William Peter Blatty that inspired a blockbuster film by the same name.

It's an incredible con job when you think about it, to believe something now in exchange for something after death. Even corporations with their reward systems don't try to make it posthumous.
-Gloria Steinem

The many other popular execution methods, some which prevailed for only limited periods of time, included being slowly choked to death or "garroted," the standard age-old method of hanging; "immurement," a term indicating that the individual has been sentenced to die in solitary confinement; and death in chambers filled with poisonous gas—used for a limited time in some states.

As if these weren't already enough to boggle the mind, some societies or cultures have eagerly impaled the condemned with sharp poles, sometimes entering the anus and eventually exiting the mouth. Often, rather than merely getting jabbed through the back or front of their bodies, these victims are slowly pierced through the central mass of their bodies.

Impalements occasionally were performed at the height of intense public strife, such as amid rebellions, wars or religious persecutions. Sometimes after completing the deed the killers "shamed" the dead by leaving their copses on display in public places.

The poles by which they had been impaled were lodged into the ground, the corpse displayed in an erect position with the pole visibly protruding into the anus and exiting from the chest, shoulders, the nape of the neck, head or mouth. These displays also were supposedly arranged to block any chance the dead might have to exit from their graves.

In various sections of the Africa continent, some conquerors from Portugal, Spain and the Netherlands used impalement to punish slaves or to dominate indigenous tribes. The executioners used long metal or wood stakes affixed to hooks to penetrate the body's central mass. Some accounts claim executioners used stakes with rounded tips in order to pass by vital organs, thereby to avoid damaging them during the piercing process.

I'm not afraid of death, but I resent it. I think it's unfair and irritating.

-Viggo Mortensen

Thanks largely to this factor, when performed as intended, an impaled person dies a few hours, and even up to three days after their bodies are fully pierced, according to a wide variety of published scholarly accounts.

Some cultures that imposed death by impalement strived to achieve the slowest, most painful death possible by pushing the stake close to the spine—a method deemed the most likely pathway for avoiding vital organs.

The precise pathway through the body was sometimes left to the discretion of the executioner.

Various written accounts from many cultures tell of victims writhing and screaming in pain after being impaled—begging for people to kill them. Numerous other accounts tell of impaled people engaging in conversations, their full-body piercing so expertly done that they were able to drink or even eat while awaiting certain death.

Documentation left by witnesses indicate that 8,000 Janis who refused to convert to Shaivism were impaled in a mass execution in India, killed under orders by King Koon Pandiyan in the Maduri Massacre 700 years after Christ. Witnesses reported that many of the executed lived for a number of hours after being impaled.

During the Ottoman Empire over a period of hundreds of years thousands of condemned criminals were successfully and skillfully vertically impaled. These victims remained alive after the procedure, only to be slowly roasted over open flames—the stake used to pierce their bodies then utilized as a barbecue pit, slowly roasted the victims alive. Thomas Smart Hughes, a British historian who visited Greece and Albania in 1812-13, witnessed many of these impalement and roasting executions—which sometimes ended with the condemned being skinned alive.

Less than 200 years ago in 1821, following the Siege of Tripolista the Greeks impaled thousands of people before slowly burning them alive.

According to eyewitness accounts from the 1600s, longitudinal piercing often was started through the rectum or vagina, or through another hole or wound inflicted in order to commence the execution—such as using a knife, hatchet, ax or a razor to make an incision through the sacrum, a large triangular bone at the base of the spine.

Numerous reports indicate that salve was sometimes used to stop or prevent excessive bleeding during and immediately after this initial cut. Shortly before execution, the condemned were usually undressed and forced to lie down face-down on their bellies.

About Death

I couldn't have foreseen all the good things that have followed my mother's death. The renewed energy, the surprising sweetness of grief. The tenderness I feel for strangers on walkers. The deeper love I have for my siblings and friends. The desire to play the mandolin. The gift of a visitation.

-Mary Schmich

To prevent excessive struggling that might hamper the executioner's work, various assistants would tie the condemned person's hands behind the back. Numerous witnesses reported in their various written accounts that at this point additional assistants would hold the victim's legs spread-eagle in opposite directions.

Pierre Belon, a French naturalist, diplomat and writer who witnessed many impalement executions in the 1500s while traveling extensively through Palestine, Arabia, Egypt and Asia Minor, wrote that numerous assistants sometimes tied the limbs to poles stuck into the ground—shortly before the execution stake was inserted vertically through the entire body.

In at least one instance, Belon wrote, a condemned person was hoisted into the air using pulleys before summarily being lowered onto an iron pole that already had been erected. In addition, various historians claim that prior to impalements the execution stakes sometimes were covered with grease in order to enable the entire implement to slide more easily through the entire body.

Then, once the stake had been initially inserted through the anus, vagina or the lower-body wound, the executioner used a mallet to steadily hammer the stake through the entire body cavity. The executioner's team of assistants also held various sections of the condemned person's body in order to help ensure that the stake's tip remained inside the main cavity until finally exiting from the head, neck or chest.

Ideally, the stake exited through the mouth while the person remained alive, left helplessly shaking while remaining alive for several hours.

James W. Forsythe, M.D., H.M.D.

Additional documentation indicates that a different method was used, as assistants gradually pulled the condemned person's legs apart could be successfully completed in a much slower and more methodical process.

Most executioners and their masters reportedly desired a full impalement exiting through the head. Yet sometimes either by design or a miscalculation the tip of the stake exited from the upper torso, the neck, shoulder or chest.

Such executions were not confined to criminals. In 1789, the explorer Captain John Adams wrote of his revulsion at witnessing an annual ritual in Lagos—now Nigeria in Africa—where a young virgin female was chosen for impalement. Adams wrote that the culture's men became cheerful at the festivities conducted to please the gods.

As recently as the early 1800s witnesses including Samuel Gridley Howe of Massachusetts, saw numerous impalement executions in Greece during the Greek Revolution. Howe reported that immediately following full insertions the stakes are not always vertically erected on the ground. When this happens, the victims sometimes writhed in pain during their final minutes of life.

All interest in disease and death is only another expression of interest in life.

-Thomas Mann

The many other seemingly countless forms of execution have included: "keelhauling," the dragging of the condemned in the water along the keel of a boat; poisoning, via lethal injection or ingested in a variety of forms; and the pendulum, which slowly swung over an extended period of time before slicing into the condemned person.

The Persians developed the "scaphism" execution method, in which executioners secured the naked condemned person inside two narrow rowing boats or hallowed-out tree trunks. Then, the executioner forced the person to drink lots of honey and milk.

These foods in turn forced the individual to expel diarrhea or extremely loose bowel movements. Meantime, the killers rubbed additional honey on the person's limbs.

This process invariably attracted streams of insects, including flies, wasps and bees. At this point the executioners leave their victim exposed to the elements or floating in a stagnant pond. The person continues to defecate within the container in which they're confined. Massive amounts of insects converge, eating the live person's flesh.

This in turn interrupts the blood supply in various areas of the body, which become gangrenous. The insect's continuous daily feedings at the infected and dying flesh causes the victim excruciating, non-stop pain.

To prolong the torture the executioners continue to force-feed the victim with generous amounts of honey and milk. Many victims became delirious for days, some dying from septic shock, starvation and exposure to the elements.

I can choose to accelerate my disease to an alcoholic death or incurable insanity, or I can choose to live within my thoroughly human condition.

- Mercedes McCambridge

Still commonly used even today in various cultures, death by gunshot is a quick death for the condemned. Most die via firing squad, while some nations such as China inflict a single shot to the neck or head.

Those who die in solitary confinement mentioned earlier often succumb from starvation.

For a period of many thousands of years up until 1903, "slow-slicing" was a common form of execution in China. Over extended periods of time, sometimes many days or weeks, the executioner would methodically slice or chop off body parts.

This method was reserved for the worst crimes, particularly treason. Devilish executioners sometimes chose to slice away a fingertip, returning daily to slice the additional fingertips—one-by-one, always leaving the victim alive to suffer.

Beginning many years after such execution rituals began, authorities started allowing the administering of opium as an act of mercy, but also to keep the person conscious and at least somewhat pain-free for as long as possible.

Cuts to the arms, legs and chest were eventually followed by limb amputations.

When scheduled properly, the executioner steadily and methodically progressed in daily cutting until the point when slices of flesh were extracted from the body. The final strike often came via stabbing the heart or decapitation.

Some researchers have argued that such executions were not a "death by a thousand cuts" as many people have wrongly believed. Instead, massive blood loss invariably caused many to lose consciousness before they eventually died.

Liberty for wolves is death to the lambs.
                                             -Isaiah Berlin

All this cruelty imposed by diverse cultures throughout history worldwide sometimes can be put into clear perspective, partly for some terminally ill people now striving to cope with their current situation.

Unlike most people who have been directly or indirectly sacrificed by their governments, religions or countrymen, cancer victims at least were able to "live out their natural lives"—most into adulthood.

Much of the time while still healthy we fail to put the limited time of our own lives into a grand perspective. Remember, as indicated earlier, each individual comprises just one of the more than seven billion people now alive.

About Death

As the once-common practices of blatantly sacrificing people gradually faded during the past several hundred years, people have a greater opportunity to learn and to appreciate the deep, abiding and naturally important intrinsic value of each human life.

Anyone terminally ill at this moment, if their cognitive abilities remain viable, can strive to take a few months to ponder how they fit within the grand scope of our universe.

Even among those of us who fail to or refuse to believe in religious teachings, to say that "life has no meaning" would be to ignore the fact that we are here now, we have a presence within this world, and that when we die a void gets left behind. The essence of your own uniqueness, the good part of you, shall always remain—no matter what.

Tears are sometimes an inappropriate response to death. When a life has been lived completely honestly, completely successfully, or just completely, the correct response to death's perfect punctuation mark is a smile.

-Julie Burchill

Chapter 21

Death Customs

The vast majority of people seem to give little or no thought to this continual, non-stop blaze of information about death—until learning they have a terminal illness.

Suddenly, they no longer are mentally able to block the ultimately inescapable question regarding what death might mean to them and to their families.

Death has instilled vastly different unique customs, varying throughout history in sharply diverse nations worldwide. The topic emerges as a hot and unavoidable subject, seeping into religion, mythology, entertainment, literature and ethical issues.

Some cultures such as across North America have condemned suicide as being sinful and unethical. Conversely, various Far Eastern cultures have viewed intentional self-destruction as a righteous and much-esteemed way to retain honor.

At various points in time, perhaps even more today than in the past, many countries additionally have had vastly different laws or customs allowing or prohibiting executions.

Liberty for wolves is death to the lambs.
-Isaiah Berlin

Particularly in the North American culture custom and common law dictates that dead bodies be disposed of—or at least put in a preserved state—soon after death.

Common disposal methods across the continent include

placement in crypts, burial with the body almost-always in a coffin, or burning the corpse via cremation.

Ancient cultures, particularly in Northern Africa countries like Egypt and the Middle East often placed bodies in a sarcophagus, box-like stone receptacles for storing corpses.

The use of crypts, concealed private areas for burying human remains, has been most dominant in Asia and Europe, while less common in North America.

Crypts sometimes contain burial vaults or tombs to store human remains. These are sometimes located at cemeteries, but also at public buildings or churches.

Some cultures including within parts of North America people call crypts "mausoleums," usually designed specifically as elaborate places for storing human remains. These sometimes are designed as "tombs," or "sepulchers," smaller structures than mausoleums while storing just one or a handful of dead bodies.

Consciousness after death demonstrates the possibility of consciousness operating independently of the body.

-Sanislav Grof

Sometimes religious customs or family traditions mandate the use of burial vaults, brick-lined spaces underground for one or more burials. These structures usually are family-owned, designated as eternal storage places for a limited number of relatives.

A much less frequent place for burying or storing the dead are church monuments, located in yards adjacent to houses or buildings of worship. Some religious leaders or relatives of the dead build church monuments above graves.

The numerous other above- or under-ground structures for placing the dead in various cultures have included: hypogeum tombs in ancient Egypt; "kokh," rectangular, sloping spaces cut into large natural rocks; "mausolea," commonly called ancient pyramids in a variety of cultures; and "megalithic tombs," sometimes called "chamber tombs," covered by earthen mounds, much more common in pre-historic times.

Another fairly large structure prevalent in ancient times—but rarely or never built today—were "rock-cut tombs." These were carved out of rock, some extensive.

The ancient culture of India built Samadhi or shrines to people or saints deemed sacred in the Hindu religion.

Pay mind to your own life, your own health, and wholeness. A bleeding heart is of no help to anyone if it bleeds to death.
-Frederick Buechner

Throughout history numerous cultures and particularly sailors were forced to dispose of the dead in the only available natural places available—at or near where people died.

Vikings between 800 and 1,100 years after Christ often disposed of the corpses of their leaders or comrades by putting the remains on boats, which were then burned.

Burials at sea by dropping a wrapped corpse into water became necessary among sailors, pirates, navies and private citizens—particularly during wartime. The location of a ship sometimes prevented the timely shipment of body back home, before extensive decomposition would begin; preservation methods are usually unavailable on board.

I'm more afraid of marriage than death.
-Shakira

Within the United States, the funeral business—typically called the "death care industry"—encompasses an extensive variety of services and products.

About Death

Some unofficial estimates list the annual overall revenues of the funeral industry at many billions of dollars. The services, some mandated by law or by tradition, typically include standard burials and cremations.

The related services, products or facilities, most requiring at least some form of payment, include funeral homes, funeral or memorial services, cemeteries, and crematoria, plus the sellers or producers of coffins and headstones.

Additionally, the many other related services or products might include flowers, gifts for the bereaved, food prepared by relatives and friends, or catering for wakes, and the printing of informational fliers distributed during funeral or memorial services.

The costs shoot up even higher, sometimes reaching many hundreds or thousands of dollars, for mourners of the deceased including relatives and friends who choose to travel to the services. Lodging in motels, hotels or other facilities adds to these costs.

For surviving relatives or for the dead person's estate, some or all the costs are covered by burial insurance. When such policies have not been purchased beforehand by the dead person or the deceased individual's family, the funeral expenses are typically paid for by surviving relatives or from funds obtained from the dead person's estate.

You cannot schedule death.

-Paloma Faith

State or local governments usually require embalming when the body has been designated for placement underground, in a tomb or vault.

With techniques varying among different cultures, embalming involves the removal of certain body fluids and the implementation of specific chemical compounds—all done with the intention of preserving the remains or slowing the decomposition process.

Particularly within the United States, much of the embalming process is done as part of a multi-phase process that attempts to make the body appear acceptable for display at funerals.

Besides concentrating on bodily fluids, embalmers pay careful attention to grooming the corpse and to attire—often provided by the deceased person's surviving relatives.

Highly trained embalmers proficient at meeting government- and industry-imposed regulations use a variety of chemicals, disinfectants and sanitizers. Mixtures vary worldwide to create embalming fluid, depending on specific cultures.

Your ego can become an obstacle to your work. If you start believing in your own greatness, it is the death of your creativity.

-Marina Abramovic

According to numerous public reports, within the United States embalming fluid usually contains various solvents plus wetting agents, ethanol, glutaraldehyde, and formaldehyde. Besides making the viewable areas of the body including the hands and head appear lifelike, most modern embalming procedures strive to at least temporarily decelerate the body's overall natural decomposition process.

Yet the vast majority of embalmed bodies eventually decompose, the flesh eventually degrading into dust and the bones gradually disappearing over time.

For those who are buried, decomposition sometimes accelerates when moisture seeps into a coffin underground or when insects, worms and rodents invade the casket.

Strangely, the vast majority of mourners have what some funeral industry professionals call an "unrealistic expectation" that a body should look precisely as the person did while alive. Nonetheless, embalmers and morticians strive to achieve the lifelike appearance by administering make-up after inserting embalming fluids.

Depending on the circumstances in which the person died, embalmers sometimes are delayed in commencing their work. Certain circumstances dictate that their job must wait until after a government employee conducts an autopsy, to determine the circumstances and the likely cause of death.

Many jurisdictions requires autopsies if the person was found dead while not under constant medical care, or when the individual died under mysterious circumstances while not suffering from any known serious ailments or diseases.

Death is an endless night so awful to contemplate that it can make us love life and value it with such passion that it may be the ultimate cause of all joy and all art.
-Paul Theroux

In instances where the body has been autopsied, embalmers sometimes choose to employ various procedures that these professionals don't typically use for "standard deaths while under medical care."

These additional procedures designed to help assure bodily preservation or to delay composition are sometimes deemed necessary because autopsies temporarily or permanently remove certain organs—while disrupting the circulatory system.

In addition, some families or governments might request or demand long-term preservation of a body. Such procedures are intended to keep the corpse as appearing natural much longer than the carcasses that undergo standard embalming.

A much different and highly specialized technique is used for the preservation of bodies that have been designated for use by doctors or by medical students. This procedure focuses on the long-term preservation of the flesh, rather than striving to make a corpse appear presentable for a funeral. This lacks unnecessary dyes and perfumes.

James W. Forsythe, M.D., H.M.D.

Also coming into play are a wide variety of differing rules and customs that involve embalming, dictated by belief systems from around the world. Many religions such as most Christian branches and the Church of Jesus Christ of Latter Day Saints do not discourage or prohibit embalming.

But some practitioners of paganism discourage the process because they want the body to revert into its natural state within the earth as readily and as quickly as Mother Nature dictates. Numerous other religions discourage or prohibit embalming. Practitioners of Zoroastrianism, an ancient Persian religion, want the body to decompose in natural conditions such as in a Tower of Silence while exposed to the elements.

Survivors who embrace traditional Jewish law are prohibited from allowing the deceased to be embalmed, while burial is preferred within one day after death.

We are not our own. We do not belong to ourselves. But we have been purchased with a dear price. We have cost an immense sum, even the sufferings and death of the Son of God.

-Ellen G. White

National governments and massive amounts of mourners from some countries have required the long-term embalming of famous or widely revered public figures.

Celebrities, government officials or religious icons highly preserved for non-stop public display for a period of years have included: Joseph Stalin, the de-facto leader of the Soviet government from the 1920s until his death in the early 1950s; Vladimir Lenin, a Russian communist, Marxist and revolutionary who led that country from 1917 until his death in 1924; Abraham Lincoln, 16th President of the United States; Eva Perón, First Lady of Argentina from 1946 until her death in 1952; and Rosalia Lombardo, a Sicilian child who died at age 2 from influenza in 1920, whose embalmed body remains so well preserved that the

About Death

corpse remains on display at the famed Capuchin catacombs of Palermo in Sicily.

But even the most famous embalming efforts fail to eternally stall or prevent decomposition. The famous mummified body of little Rosalia has finally begun to discolor, according to a 2009 article and photo in "National Geographic" magazine.

Thirty-six years after his 1865 assassination, President Lincoln's body was exhumed in 1901, when witnesses reported his body's features remained remarkably recognizable.

Some decisions to embalm famous people have become controversial. Via request from officials or from her family, authorities in France embalmed the body of Diana, Princess of Wales, in August 1997 after her death in a Paris auto accident. The embalming sparked a conspiracy theory among people who claim that the procedure has prevented an adequate official government autopsy of her body.

It is just as idiotic to say there is no life after death as it is to say there is one.
-Jeanne Moreau

Chapter 22

Burning Bodies

Cremation reigns as the other popular, most-used method of body disposal in the United States, while also dominant in many cultures in many other nations.

The burning of dead bodies prevails in many religions within India, particularly Hinduism. Numerous India cultures burn bodies in open-air pyres, particularly at locations where such events are widely accepted—often in accordance with the rules of certain religions.

Many other countries widely embrace the custom and traditions of cremation, such as Bali and Thailand.

Within the religious realm, Catholics historically have discouraged cremation, partly because the human body is considered holy or sacred. Catholics in medieval Europe banned the practice. But since the Middle Ages many of the faithful within this church have begun to allow the practice.

Starting in 1997, the Catholic Church officially began allowing the remains of cremations—technically called "cremains"—to be at the Funeral Lithurgy This "inult" or privilege was granted by the Vatican's Congregation for Devine Worship and the Discipline of the Sacraments.

Particularly since the 1870s Protestants have been much more welcoming of cremation than Catholics. Simultaneously some branches of the Eastern Orthodox Church have opposed cremation. The LDS Church had discouraged cremation, but recently published specifics on how families should dress the deceased prior to cremation. Many sectors of Judaism have discouraged or prohibited cremation.

Failure too is a form of death.
-Graham Greene

Historical documentation and archaeological discoveries have indicated that some cultures have cremated the dead as recently as 20,000 years ago. One of the oldest known discoveries of the partially cremated remains of a body were found in Australia.

More recently, according to published reports some cultures or societies in Persia began cremating their dead about 3,000 years before Christ. The Greeks buried all dead people until about 1,200 years before Christ when various communities began occasionally cremating the dead.

During the final thousand years before Jesus' birth numerous societies across Europe added cremation to their body-disposal options. Despite the spread of this process, some religions began complaining about each other decisions regarding cremation.

Religious leaders in many European cultures criticized any spiritual belief system in which living people were sacrificed in fires or living people who chose to die that way.

Even so, cremation became increasingly common in the ancient Greek and Roman empires, although not the only body-disposal method.

Living with the immediacy of death helps you sort out your priorities in life. It helps you to live a less trivial life.
-Sogyal Rinpoche

The cremation of the dead suddenly accelerated on an industrial scale in Germany during World War II in the late 1930s and early 1940s. Nazis from Adolph Hitler's notorious Third Reich cremated the bodies of slaughtered Jews by the millions.

James W. Forsythe, M.D., H.M.D.

Devilish German military leaders ordered and supervised the construction of giant crematories; the most notorious of these enormous furnaces were at six human-extermination camps.

According to some Nazi documentation published in 1996, the Third Reich's crematorium at Birkenau in Poland cremated 6,000 bodies daily.

More than 60 years later, a lack of necessary resources forced authorities in numerous countries to simultaneously burn thousands of bodies.

The impromptu outdoor funeral pyres were lit after a tsunami killed 300,000 people in a single day in many countries including several African nations, Malaysia, Indonesia, Thailand and India.

People who are sick or who have been sick, or have come close to death have a lot to say—and they want you to hear it.

-Anna Deavere Smith

Sociologists say that cremation is chosen by many people for a variety of personal and economic reasons. Many people dislike the alternative, the slow decomposition process—which they consider revolting.

Also, particularly if done with planning and commitment, the overall costs of cremation can be significantly lower than for traditional funerals that include caskets.

These costs can vary among states and nations. But in general, the expense for a simple cremation in the United States can be as low as several hundred dollars or $400-$700 at most—particularly if the person makes an advance payment while alive.

This compares to thousands of dollars for caskets, plus the rental of funeral homes, hearse services and any payment as a tithing to a church representative such as a pastor or a preacher. Partly for these reasons, some people who intend to be cremated also decide to ask that no formal funeral or celebration of life be held.

About Death

Urns can cost hundreds of dollars, sometimes sold by funeral homes or crematoriums. Survivors who choose to side-step such costs sometimes "cremains" delivered in plastic wrappings and cardboard boxes.

All along, some national, state or municipal governments required that corpses be cremated only while inside a container such as a casket. However, some surviving relatives or deceased people prior to their deaths decide that the body should be engulfed in flames while inside the cheapest allowable container, such as a cardboard box.

"If it was my father or mother, I wouldn't want to go in such a cheap way," some funeral home personnel have been known to say to grieving mourners who must make a decision. Such words spoken in kind tones often motivate survivors to choose more expensive options. This is partly why some people choose to make that decision when arranging and paying for their own future cremations and for the related services that entails.

Knowing how to die is knowing how to live. What is death anyway? It's the outcome of life.
        -Jeanne Moreau

Additional motivation for choosing cremation sometimes stems from the fact that this process often simplifies the entire process for survivors.

Some people like the fact that cremains can be stored in boxes or urns, and the remains can be legally scattered in the natural environment. This also cuts down on ground needed fill cemeteries.

Yet for those who choose cremation but want a spot for people to visit their remains, some burial facilities provide cremation plots or columbarium—structures used for the storage of cinerary urns.

The ancient Roman culture was among the first to construct

columbarium buildings. Today, some of these structures are built at or shipped to cemeteries.

Other increasingly prevalent sites for columbarium include crematoria in major world-renowned cities including Paris and London. Numerous churches also have begun permitting the construction of or the additions of this feature in their facilities.

Death is a sanction of everything the storyteller can tell. He has borrowed his authority from death.

-Walter Benjamin

Despite the apparent ease, cost savings and simplifications that cremation can provide, some people have insisted that this process endangers the environment.

According to various publications, critics have alleged that the body-burning process subjects the atmosphere to certain contaminants.

The cremation process technically does not result in ashes from the body's flesh. Instead, the flesh converts into gasses that go into the atmosphere. Some nations or municipalities in Europe require that the cremation process use devices to filter mercury and other potentially harmful contaminants.

Some critics also allege that concrete or other linings that surround traditional caskets collectively take up too much space on the earth.

Without fullness of experience, length of days is nothing. When fullness of life has been achieved, shortness of days is nothing. That is perhaps why the young usually have so little fear of death; they live by intensities that the elderly have forgotten.

-Lewis Mumford

Chapter
23

Funeral Rituals

Archaeologists report that for the past 300,000 years humans have adopted a wide variety of funeral customs and procedures. Today's traditions are of huge importance to the more than 7 billion living people who will be celebrated or mourned after death.

Depending on their cultural traditions and religious rules, funerals in some regions can last from only a matter of a few minutes to a period stretching over several days.

Many people cherish funerals in part for the cultural significance of such ceremonies, often considered as appropriate remembrances of the dead. Other living individuals dread the thought of attending.

Religions and churches have their own sacred rites, utterances and symbols for funerals, processes that many people who attend fail to understand.

As dictated by each church and the degree of formality requested by the grieving family or the deceased person, much of the time the event can be formal or at least somewhat informal.

You haven't lost anything when you know where it is. Death can hide but not divide.
-Vance Havner

Buddhists have a variety of customs, largely dependant on the region where the person has lived "his most recent life."

Remember, as indicated earlier, this religion or belief system perceives this lifetime as temporary before the soul naturally and predictably transitions into additional lives—a continual learning process until ultimately achieving Nirvana.

Under most sectors of the Christianity the burial process involves ecclesiastical rites, meaning that the event follows specific criteria as specified by the church. The priest, preacher or reverent focuses on salvation under the church's guidance and leadership, coupled with how we must behave in life in order to earn entrance into heaven.

Particularly until about a century ago, Christian clergy would often start the proceedings by first visiting the home of the dead person—sprinkling the corpse there with Holy Water. From there accompanied by clergy a coffin containing the body was taken to the church.

Although this home-visiting phase is done much less frequently today, many of the other traditions held by most Christian churches remain generally or loosely similar to funeral rites performed long ago.

Common funeral ceremonies depend on the degree of formality arranged. Features range from prayers, a requiem mass, an absolution asking God to spare the person from purgatory; and eventually a graveside ceremony.

I very much faced my mother's death with hard, arduous and time-consuming labor. The more I would do, the less I would feel.
                                                              -Rufus Wainwright

Additional funeral traditions often used in ceremonies of the Orthodox or Eastern Catholic Church include: "last kiss," where mourners give the corpse a final kiss; a "memory eternal," words recited slowly three times during the funeral or memorial service as a remembrance of God rather than of the living; and a "divine liturgy," which is believed to transcend time and worldly things.

Islam has numerous specific rituals, such as positioning the deceased so that the head faces Mecca, bathing the body, enshrouding the corpse with white cotton or linen cloth, burying the body and saying prayers.

The Sikh faith closely associates birth and death, the soul's progression in a journey to God. Sikh people discourage loud crying and wailing at funerals. After being washed and dressed, the body is taken on the day of cremation to a home or Gurdwara. Participants recite scriptures intended to instill courage and consolation.

Participants then take the body to a cremation site after this ceremony, which usually lasts 30 minutes to one hour. During the cremation, participants can make final speeches or sing Shabads. Later after the funeral pyre cools, participants collect the cremains before throwing them into the Punjab—one of India's five primary rivers.

Buy a steak for another player after the game, but don't even speak to him on the field. Get out there and beat them to death.

-Leo Durocher

A blend of the Buddhist and Shintō faiths is often used for funerals in Japan. While generally following these faiths, the rites focus on the dead person's passage through life.

Throughout the Philippines, mourners at funerals often embrace or participate using a wide variety of traditional, religious and cultural beliefs. Lots of the sources indicate that the diverse funeral traditions Filipinos use were first brought to their nation by colonialists and various religions.

Across Europe and North America, a long-held tradition continued by many religions and families involves a scheduled "viewing" of the dead person—sometimes called "calling hours." These are sometimes preceded by obituary notices in printed newspapers or online, asking that mourners give to certain charities, organizations or surviving family members in "lieu of flowers."

The viewing of the dead person often takes place in a funeral home. Some cultures including regions of Scotland prefer to display the body in the individual's personal residence. These gatherings are sometimes called memorial services or "celebrations of life." Relatives of the deceased often speak about the person.

At the actual funeral, relatives or friends of the dead person—and on rare occasions, celebrities or notable individuals—are chosen to give eulogies. These often entail personal stories about the individual, sometimes drawing laughter or tears.

My father I liked, but it was only after his death that I got to know him by writing the play.
                              -Hugh Leonard

A wide variety of relatives, friends and acquaintances gather for a wake or luncheon after the funeral, often following tradition or via request of family mourners, or to fulfill the dead person's wishes.

Wakes sometimes evolve into wild rowdy affairs, while many such celebrations remain intentionally sedate and rather solemn affairs where most people chat softly.

This is a part of the overall funeral process that many mourners dread, particularly family members. Some relatives feel as if they're forced into an uncomfortable situation, where they must converse with relatives that they dislike or who lack mutual respect.

Some religious leaders and psychologists say these unwanted reunions sometimes provide an opportunity for at least temporary reconciliation. In essence, due to the death the caused the wake, a once-sour relationship might have an opportunity to rekindle.

About Death

Accepted cultural traditions in each country sometimes dictate who can or should attend certain funeral-related events. Some traditions dictate that the closest relatives at a graveside service should wear formal clothing. This might tend to irritate some people upon seeing relatives who would dare show up in very casual attire.

Filled with grief from the loss of their husbands or lovers, some women wear veils that hide their facial expressions. Many mourners follow a tradition of signing a guest book, which the deceased person's closest relatives often keep as a remembrance.

I think the minute you mention death, people run for the hills—unless it's heavy metal. People do not like death.

-Rufus Wainwright

Some funerals are kept extremely small and very private, open only to invited relatives and close friends. This is sometimes done in order to keep the news media away from mourning services that involve living or deceased celebrities, or as a private matter due to the death of an infant.

Other reasons for insisting on privacy sometimes include trying to avoid a sense of notoriety, particularly if the dead person was a convicted killer or a criminal.

In addition, some families collectively find themselves wanting to avoid huge crowds, particularly after the sudden and unexpected death from an accident leaves them in a state of mental shock.

Additionally, the number of participants might be kept intentionally low in order to minimize expenses. Occasionally under such circumstances, and even when finances aren't considered a primary concern, some relatives prefer to arrange for the disposal of cremains at a time that most family members consider convenient.

Conversely, some families and friends enjoy what they call a

James W. Forsythe, M.D., H.M.D.

"New Orleans-style jazz funeral," where people arrive and leave free of charge—everyone bringing at least some food for sharing, and most helping with clean-up chores afterward.

Defeat the fear of death, and welcome the death of fear.
                                                    -G. Gordon Liddy

Environmental concerns motivate some families, and even the dead person who had previously planned such an event, to plan "green funerals."

These usually are instances where the body is wrapped in a bio-degradable burial shroud, buried in a natural, non-embalmed state in order to naturally decay in a wilderness area such as a park or forest.

Many humanists believe in an afterlife. Even so, they choose to organize funerals that cherish and focus upon the dead person's life, rather than any religion.

In our increasingly tech-based, insensitive and impersonal world, "Internet funerals and visitations" also have begun in recent years. Rather than bother with the time and expense of attending an event in person, "mourners" watch briefly via live Webcasts—sometimes texting in messages about their supposed sorrow.

Funeral services for police officers and firefighters, particularly those who perished in the line of duty, often are the biggest such events in the United States. In some communities hundreds or even thousands of people take the time to attend.

Fear was absolutely necessary. Without it, I would have been scared to death.
                    -Floyd Patterson

Many mourners in the Western culture wear black clothing as a sign of their grief. The opposite holds true at East Asian funerals, where white has symbolized death for thousands of years. Yet some aspects of the West's traditions have moved into the East Asian culture, which now permits at least some darker clothing at funerals.

Vast numbers of funerals in the West in recent years have been deemed as "celebrations," but that term in East Asian nations is reserved for people who died past their mid-80s.

In South China mourners arrive giving envelopes containing money to relatives of the person who died, similar to the way relatives in the West celebrate weddings.

Even today, in West Africa common funeral traditions are much different than in the rest of the world. There, mourners usually arrive at the deceased person's home, or at the residences of that person's relatives, to see the corpse set out on the dwelling floor.

Funerals are much more expensive and elaborate in East African countries, particularly Kenya. Some mourning relatives keep the deceased person's body stored at a morgue or funeral home for extended periods, allowing sufficient time to raise the necessary funds to pay for the funeral.

Relatives of the dead in Kenya sometimes take many days off from their jobs, partly in order to spend the necessary and extensive time to prepare for a huge feast. Economists say this becomes a huge drag on the economy, where from half to three-quarters of the population earns $1 or less per day.

To be immortal is commonplace; except for man, all creatures are immortal, for they are ignorant of death; what is divine, terrible, incomprehensible, is to know that one is immortal.

-Jorge Luis Borges

Today's diverging funeral traditions on an international scale are vastly different from what most cultures engaged in following deaths thousands of years ago.

James W. Forsythe, M.D., H.M.D.

The books of Joshua, Homer and Virgil describe the disposal of bodies on large earthen mounds. Jewish people in ancient times usually lacked designated burial sites.

During primitive times, archaeologists say, the mourners of dead Greeks buried the corpses at the dwellings where the deceased people lived. Kings or royalty during those times often had the distinction of being buried in fields near the graves of relatives.

Continuing the practice started thousands of years ago in their culture, the vast majority of funerals in Greece today a casket remains open during the funeral—with the event starting in the home where the person lived. In some regions of Greece, mourners put coins in the casket as payment to prevent the god Charon from ferrying the person's soul to the underworld.

Also continuing a longtime tradition, today's surviving mourners in Greece frequently plant lots of flowers at the tombs of their beloved, partly to ensure that the deceased remain in repose.

Fear not; for the God of mercies grant a full gale and a fair entry into His kingdom, which may carry sweetly and swiftly over the bar, that you find not the rub of death.
-Donald Cargill

Thousands of years before Christ the Egyptians mummified their leaders before burial in tombs at the famed pyramids.

This process involved perhaps the first known highly intricate attempts at embalming. Only after the embalming was completed, the Pharaohs were entombed in a sarcophagus, the carved stone structures mentioned earlier.

Gradually over time the Egyptian royalty developed a system mandating that dead leaders would be entombed in several layers of coffins—many carved from alabaster. The stone Hagia Triada sarcophagus Embossed with elaborate printing painted in fresco.

Some of these historically significant artifacts are now kept safely in a British museum, far away from violent public strife in today's Egypt and Middle East.

The various collections amassed from these tombs indicate that Pharaohs and their subjects engaged in elaborate funeral preparation. In fact, the entire construction project of the pyramids served the ultimate goal of getting the ancient Egyptian leaders into the afterlife. This signifies that early in the history of humanity people from an early age were able to put great thought into their own eventual deaths, starting from a very early age.

Loss and possession, death and life are one. There falls no shadow where there shines no sun.

-Hilaire Belloc

Roman funerals were plentiful and elaborate. Relatives of the dead person often wore masks reminiscent of the individual. Morticians hired professional female mourners, plus many entertainers including magicians, dancers and mimes, all employed to participate in funeral processions.

The Roman community considered the dead person's house as tainted for the first nine days following the funeral. Then, the house was swept to remove the residence of any taint of death, and a celebration feast summarily began. Politicians in early Rome set limits on what people could do during funeral celebrations.

Much later in Scotland, perhaps starting around from 800 to 1,200 years after Christ, mourners often placed a plate on the dead person's chest. To signify the dead person's future the funeral-goers placed salt and dirt. Salt never decays and remains forever just like the soul, while the dirt returns to blend in with the rest of the earth.

A common funeral practice that reportedly occurred across much of Europe involved the hiring of mutes and professional female mourners.

The mutes, typically men, stood at the funerals—their faces

James W. Forsythe, M.D., H.M.D.

embossed with sad and mournful expressions. The hired women added to the sense of drama and grief, wailing, crying and shirking at all the appropriate times.

Constantly risking absurdity and death whenever he performs above the heads of his audience, the poet, like an acrobat, climbs on rhyme to a high wire of his own making.
                                                              -Lawrence Ferlinghetti

In more recent times, particularly during the last half of the 20th Century and into the current century, state funerals evolved into elaborate events attracting dignitaries worldwide. State funerals for major world and national leaders in the United States and in Great Britain drew much of the attention, plus in other English speaking nations as well.

Lots of these deaths generated various national days of mourning, amid intense national and international publicity and continuous TV, radio and Internet coverage. Significant state funerals have been conducted in each occupied continent.

Some of the most significant funerals to gain worldwide attention thanks partly to new telephone and telegraph technology at the time were the deaths of officials in the Republic of China in 1917 and 1929.

One of the most recent major state-sanctioned funerals in China was in 2006 following the death of Henry Fok Ying Tung, who died at age 83 after serving as Chairman of the National Committee of the Chinese People's Political Consultative Conference. His Hong Kong funeral following treatment for cancer came as the news media dubbed him as possibly the most politically powerful people in Hong Kong.

War is not the only arena where peace is done to death.
                                                              -Aung San Suu Kyi

About Death

Journalists estimated that millions of people attended the 1948 funeral in India of Mahatma Gandhi following his assassination, widely considered the "father" of that nation. Other India funerals receiving International attention were for: Indira Gandhi, assassinated by two of her bodyguards in 1984 while she served as the third prime minister of India; Jawaharal Neru, the first prime minister of India, following his death of natural causes in 1964; and La Bahadur Shastri, the second prime minister of India, after dying of an apparent heart attack in 1966.

Elsewhere state funerals attracting extensive media coverage occurred in Cambodia, the Philippines and Singapore. The extensive TV coverage, resulting in nightly news reports in other nations, enabled people worldwide to learn about the vastly different funeral cultures performed in other countries.

At the invitation of other governments, world leaders attended many funeral services of heads of state from other nations. These gatherings may have been used at least partly in an effort to solidify relations among European countries that had been allies or enemies in World War II.

Improved communication systems and faster travel methods in the 1950s and beyond increased the ability of multiple countries to simultaneously mourn the dead.

For instance, in 1982 TV viewers in the United States and elsewhere got their first live, vivid broadcasts from the House of Unions in Moscow during the state funeral of Leonid Brezhnev. He had served as Secretary General of the Communist Party of the Soviet Union's Central Committee from 1964 until his death.

People worldwide for the first time saw the embalmed, black-suited body of a Soviet leader, the Russian military guard, and numerous communist symbols at the funeral site.

It's not life or death, it's a game at the end of a game there is going to be a winner and a loser.

-Bernhard Langer

James W. Forsythe, M.D., H.M.D.

From the United States, some of the most sensational and instantaneous worldwide TV coverage came during state funeral proceedings for President John F. Kennedy, assassinated in November 1963. Kennedy became the fourth assassinated U.S. president to have a state funeral in Washington, D.C., the first with instantaneous international news media coverage.

Perhaps more than any other state funeral before this in any nation, Kennedy's death resulted in a gathering where people worldwide shared the experience and grief process involving a single killing.

Following a rapid planning process of just three days, Kennedy's funeral Requiem Mass was celebrated at the Cathedral of St. Matthew the Apostle in Washington, D.C., on Nov. 25, 1963. Soon afterward, he was initially buried in a small plot in Arlington National Cemetery; four years later authorities moved his body to a permanent plot and memorial in the same complex.

His assassinated brother, U.S. Senator Robert Francis Kennedy, was buried near him in a small plot during intense, live worldwide TV coverage in June 1968. Another brother, U.S. Senator Edward M. Kennedy, was buried at Arlington after dying of brain cancer in August 2009, also interred during extensive live TV coverage.

It is love, not reason, that is stronger than death.

-Thomas Mann

Chapter 24
Death in Modern and Historical Cultures

Death has profoundly impacted every populated culture worldwide, everything from literature, poetry, films and stage plays, to TV and the Internet.

Starting long ago various cultural traditions impacted everything from who would take possession of a body to permissible songs or artifacts commemorating the person.

Grief and morning become an inescapable factor among survivors, as mourners struggle to mentally cope with change. Some cultures discourage mental health counseling, insisting that survivors should seek guidance from their churches.

In almost every culture, mourners often experience extreme grief and depression, particularly upon the sudden, unexpected death of a close relative—particularly a child.

Bereavement becomes particularly challenging for people who have few, if any, relatives or close friends. Besides help from their churches or mental health professionals, they sometimes seek comfort from literature, poems and movies involving death.

You can cry about death, and very properly so, your own as well as anybody else's. But it's inevitable, so you better grapple with it, and cope and be aware that not only is it inevitable, but it has always been inevitable, if you see what I mean.

-David Attenborough

Many societies, particularly local communities in the United States, have various support groups where grieving survivors can share stories about their personal grief.

Much of the time, but not always, the sense of personal loss and heartache gradually fades at least somewhat over a period of months or years. Yet some mourners experience intense grief and heartache due to the loss of a loved one, for the remainder of their lives.

"He literally died of a broken heart," becomes a common statement among survivors, describing a person who died soon after the death of a loved one.

The ability and the natural tendency of people to deeply, fully and wholly love each other can become profound and unstoppable. For many the mere thought of striving to endure through life without a cherished departed loved one becomes unbearable.

The suicide rate among U.S. military veterans of the wars in Iraq and Afghanistan has continued to spiral upward. Some analysts blame the aftermath of post traumatic stress, coupled with mental anguish over the combat deaths of their beloved fellow soldiers.

Lots of cultures strongly encourage friends, relatives and acquaintances of the dead to attend funerals as a "common courtesy" to the departed person's family. Having lots of friends around to provide comfort and at least temporary companionship can go a long way toward helping the psyche heal.

As indicated earlier, this is among primary reasons why I'm among health care professionals who strongly believe that merely grieving via text messages and the Internet is detrimental to mental health among survivors.

The only religious way to think about death is as part and parcel of life.
                                                                    -Thomas Mann

About Death

Another critical factor involves the settlement of the person's estate, even among the poor, middle-class and financially wealthy.

Disputes over who should get the cash, securities holdings or personal belongings of a dead person can wreak havoc on families, relationships and civility among relatives.

Remember, as stated earlier, I never tell my advanced Stage IV cancer patients to "get your affairs in order." Yet common sense dictates that all adults, whether healthy or ill, should make advance arrangements by completing a legal "last will and testament."

When you die, do you want the government to get everything that you've earned and amassed, or for relatives to bicker over your belongings?

Some lawyers indicate that no person can stipulate or guarantee 100-percent what will happen to their possessions after the die. Yet planning for the disbursement of property can go a long way to ensuring that your wishes are fulfilled.

Most state and national governments specify what will happen to a person's estate after death if the individual had failed to complete a legal will beforehand. These laws usually specify which surviving relatives have an initial right to property.

Without a will, and even in cases where the dead person had completed such a document, surviving relatives claiming a right to some or all of the belongings can drag on the court proceedings for many months or even years.

Only a legal professional can reliably give advice on how to complete a last will and testament or ways to manage the probate process. So, if you are healthy or ill today, whatever your personal situation you should visit a lawyer as soon as possible to help ensure that your estate—whether large or small—is disbursed in accordance with your wishes.

Death has always been a prominent place in my mind. There are times when I think someone might kill me.
                                                          -**Dennis Rodman**

James W. Forsythe, M.D., H.M.D.

Another highly controversial issue worldwide involves abortion.

Particularly in the United States, "pro-life" advocates strongly oppose abortion while arguing that such procedures are the outright murder of unborn children.

Conversely, supporters of abortion focus their own argument on the "need for family planning" and also "the right of women to make their own personal health choices."

The opponents of abortion call such statements as pure hogwash, a lame and unjustifiable excuse for murder of millions of babies.

On a technical level, abortion involves the termination of a pregnancy, removing the fetus or embryo from the womb prior to birth.

A whopping estimated 44 million abortions are performed worldwide every year, according to "The Lancet," published in 2012. If true, this means—from the perception of anti-abortion advocates—at least once every second somewhere in the world another unborn child is "murdered" or "slaughtered."

Amid this intensely controversial issue, pro-abortion advocates continue to insist that the procedure is "merely a medical procedure that involves a woman's choice."

According to a 2010 article in the "International Journal of Gynecology and Obstetrics," about four out of every ten women worldwide haves access to an abortion clinic. Many prospective mothers want induced abortions for financial reasons, claiming that they cannot afford to have children.

The laws among countries regulating or prohibiting abortion vary drastically. Some nations permit the procedure only in cases of incest and rape, or instances where pregnancy has medically been deemed as a critical endangerment to the woman's health.

My children are magical creatures and I love them to death.

                                                                                     -Jack Black

About Death

Another hot topic involving death focuses on not just people, but instead their pets. Dogs, cats and other animals often become closely bonded with their human owners.

Yet the vast majority of pets have much shorter life expectances than the people that own them. The worldwide average life expectancies for humans varies among nations, but generally seems to be at least age 75 for men and women.

This is much longer than most dogs and cats, which typically live from seven to 15 years—and occasionally even longer. As a result, many people have extreme difficulty coping with the deaths of their beloved pets after closely bonding emotionally with them.

Adding to the grief, pet owners often are faced with the need to perform euthanasia on an ailing animal, particularly a pet that seems to have little or no chance for a cure.

For many adults and especially senior citizens contemplating euthanasia for their pets becomes almost unthinkable. When the need arises, some seniors ask their adult children to drive alone with the animal to a veterinarian to perform the procedure.

Perhaps because most adult Americans get repulsed by the idea of death, lots of us prefer to call this procedure "putting the animal to sleep." Upon the loss of their beloved pets, many of their grieving owners become severely depressed.

The love expressed during life and after the pet's death sometimes becomes, in the mind of the owner at least, just as intense as the bond they feel for living and dead people. Pet cemeteries seem to be increasing in popularity on a national and worldwide scale. Some grieving owners even consider moving to different residences, feeling a need to leave the environment where they had deeply loved an animal.

In fact, the sense of loss has become so prevalent that people in some communities have launched recovery groups where individuals can share their sense of grief.

James W. Forsythe, M.D., H.M.D.

No real English gentleman, in his secret soul, was ever sorry for the death of a political economist.
                                                    -Walter Bagehot

Although briefly mentioned earlier, the propensity of war to generate death on an industrial scale also warrants additional discussion.

Countless millions of people have perished in wars during the past 5,000 years. Some historians insist that at every point in time during the past 500 years there has been at least one war raging somewhere in the world.

Military battles between nations or among large societies often occur because people are willing to fight for a cause that they believe in—or because their government leaders order them to participate. A huge percentage of those slaughtered are "innocent victims," non-combatants who happen to live within a war zone.

The methods of inflicting widespread death and destruction have accelerated while becoming increasingly "efficient" during the past century. The development of tanks, high-powered bombs, deadly gasses, military aircraft have added to the arsenal of death.

Today's collective armies of the world's greatest remaining superpowers, the United States, China and Russia, now number in the millions. This boosting of military might has occurred even though the globe is not currently engaged in an official "world war."

Political leaders insist in almost every culture and nation that the people they govern must remain in a continual state of preparedness for sudden all-out war.

Besides wounds suffered in combat, the greatest killers in many wars are diseases spread by soldiers, dysentery, starvation and exposure to the elements.

Thousands of years ago the most prevalent supposed reasons igniting wars hinged on religious differences, goals of achieving more land and seizing agricultural resources. Sociologists say these motivations seem to have evolved somewhat during the past century, often focusing on economic motivations and differences in political ideology.

Certainly if the past is used as any indication of what might occur in the future, wars will continue to erupt until the people of individual nations have the courage to defy politicians who would order them into combat—instead embracing the benefits of peace.

Giving is good, but taking is bad and brings death.

-Hesiod

The overall subject of "permissible" death on a worldwide scale becomes increasingly complex when considering changes in values involving suicide. These self-inflicted deaths can be categorized in two-categories—violent and non-violent.

With steadily increasing intensity since the early 1990s, intentional death by suicide has increased on a massive scale on the world's many battlefields.

Warriors intentionally killed themselves when attacking the enemy during World War II. Japanese airmen participated in suicide kamikaze attacks, German pilots in the Luftwaffe intentionally smashed into B-17 aircraft, and Soviet and Polish soldiers sacrificed themselves in ramming attacks.

Such tactics have been adopted by today's terrorists who kill themselves as "suicide bombers," darting into large crowds of their perceived enemies before detonation. These attacks have intensified on an international scale since terrorists hijacked four commercial aircraft on September 11, 2001, flying two of the jets filled with passengers into the former World Trade Center in New York City.

Suicide attack killers seem to value certain political ideologies or their allegiance to their comrades more than their own lives. Media reports also indicate that at least some suicide bombers in the Middle East during the past decade were recruited under a promise that their families would be paid handsomely upon their deaths.

Religious beliefs also reportedly have been a occasional motivation, a promise of a wonderful afterlife after indiscriminately sacrificing themselves to kill an enemy.

I try to write lyrics so that they won't age, which sort of leaves you with the big subjects like death, and love, and sex, and violence.

-Florence Welch

The so-called non-violent forms of suicide have also increased somewhat in the United States. Medical experts say depression has been the most frequent motivation.

But in recent years people suffering the ravages of illness or old age have cited their physical ailments as a primary motivation for killing themselves.

This process is often called "assisted suicide," where a person is intentionally euthanized with the assistance of another person.

Most states prohibit this, labeling such deaths as murder while embracing the argument that people do not have a right to kill themselves.

Many people believe that euthanasia should be allowed as an act of compassion, enabling and allowing terminally ill people suffering from tremendous physical pain to end their misery. This, they say, allows the terminally ill to die with "dignity."

But such procedures have been legalized in a small number of states, including Oregon, Washington, Montana and Vermont. Various published reports also indicate that legally assisted suicide is permissible in Belgium, Luxembourg, and the Netherlands.

It's also legal in Switzerland, but only in cases where specific circumstances make euthanasia permissible.

About Death

At least judging by various news accounts, under specific instances in other countries under court order medical facilities or relatives have been allowed to euthanize critically ill people.

On occasion some opponents of assisted suicide have complained that people requesting or demanding euthanasia are not always doing so under their own "free will." Opponents of assisted suicide contend that some victims are "talked into killing themselves," when such an act is not necessary or warranted.

Many people do not know this, but in the United States a huge percentage of hospitals and nursing home—as a matter of mercy—often speed the death process along.

Under doctors' orders or criteria set by their employers, nurses or other medical professionals often administer quantities of painkillers and other narcotics on people who are near-death—eliminating or blocking pain, while steadily turning off internal organs.

We are weak, writing is difficult, but for our own said I do not regret this journey, which has shown that Englishmen can endure hardships, help one another, and meet death with as great a fortitude as ever in the past.
-Robert Falcon Scott

Opinion polls indicate that within the United States health care professionals have sharply differing opinions on whether assisted suicide or euthanasia should be legalized.

In a 1997 survey of critical care nurses some denounced such procedures, while others insisted that euthanasia should be permitted. Some nurses viewed euthanasia to a "legitimate response to human suffering." But others who opposed making such suicides legal did so in accordance with their religious beliefs, or their opinion that some patients who want to be killed are too young to die.

Another argument against euthanasia has been labeled the

"slippery-slope" issue. These opponents worry that after patient-assisted suicide gets approved for ill people, other groups of individuals will start demanding similar rights.

These are considered as individuals potentially vulnerable to suggestions regarding their own deaths although unnecessary, including disabled people who use walkers or wheelchairs. Another worry focuses on people of low social or economic status, perhaps feeling that they should be allowed to die due to their lower "lot in life."

Intensifying the issue, some physicians reportedly worry that social prejudices against disabled people might motivate politicians to pass laws allowing such individuals to legally request euthanasia.

"Hamlet" is one of the most dangerous things ever set down on paper. All the big, unknowable questions like what it is to be a human being; the difference between sanity and insanity; the meaning of life and death; what's real and not real. All these subjects can literally drive you mad.

-Michael Sheen

A related issues involves allowing physicians to "pull the plug," when nurses take a critically ill or vegetative person off life support machines.

People can create and sign what the general public often refers to as a "living will," determined to make such decisions beforehand for themselves while still cognizant and legally able to make decisions for themselves.

Legally and technically called an "advance health care directive," these documents designate specific circumstances when the person does—or does not—want to be pulled from life support machines.

Preferring in advance to die rather than to spend the remainder of their lives in a "vegetative state," some signers of living wills decide under which conditions—if any—that they want to die. A perceived need to avoid being a burden on relatives is among frequent motivations of living will signers who choose to be taken off life support machines.

Some people with living wills worry that modern medicine is far too expensive, while also possibly prolonging life under wretchedly painful conditions stretched over lengthy periods.

Others making such a decision in advance want all available technology utilized to prolong their lives for as long as possible. Such individuals perceive themselves as fighters eager to stay alive.

The disembodied spirit is immortal; there is nothing in it that can grow old or die. But the embodied spirit sees death on the horizon as soon as its day dawns.
-Thomas Hobbes

For the first time in history since the 1980s those facing or contemplating death decide in advance whether to donate their organs after they die. In cases where such documents have not been authorized in the past, the decision on whether to donate an organ is left up to surviving relatives—often while the individual remains on life support.

The death of the entire body was once considered permanent. But the advent of organ donations can enable specific body parts to continue "living" within the bodies of others. This often enables people receiving the donations to remain alive.

The body-part transfers can include vital organs like the heart, lungs and liver. Other organs such as all or part of the eyes can significantly improve the lives of recipients.

Ironically, those desperately needing heart, lung or liver transplants are essentially praying or hoping for someone to die—so that they might live.

Ethically, many people are able to deal or cope with this issue, knowing that the individual who was shot through the head, died in a car wreck or another horrific tragedy would have died anyway. The transplantation process enables the dead to prolong the lives of the living.

Most of the time a donor's organs are extracted only after the person has been declared legally dead, such as when the brain waves have stopped. From the moment of the organs are removed health care professionals have a limited time to make the transfer.

These modern medical developments have generated a variety of ethical and moral issues that doctors, families and religious leaders never had to consider in all of previous human history.

People are scared to death of dying. I am the opposite.
-Taylor Caldwell

Another modern development has tested our ethical values even more than organ transplants. During recent decades scientists have worked feverishly to improve the study and use of cryonics. This involves freezing entire bodies or organs to extremely low temperatures, hundreds of degrees below zero.

The goal is to eventually unfreeze or slowly thaw the bodies and organs, but only after "cures" have been developed.

Numerous people in recent decades have paid to put their bodies into a deep freeze shortly after the die. These people hope to eventually be "risen from the dead," primarily after scientists have found cures for the ailments that killed them.

As a doctor, and even as a homeopath embracing natural medicines, I find the concept of bring people back to life in this way as somewhat disturbing. Yet as scientists continue their efforts to make this system workable, I also appreciate the right of people seeking these bodily freezes to seek such treatments.

Even so, some additional advances now in the works strike me as particularly repulsive; perhaps other doctors feel the same.

In recent years some world-renowned experts in the body's

nervous systems have predicted that by the 2040s medical technology will be able to transfer the head of one individual onto the neck and shoulders of another person.

Under some scenarios a person in his 80s could cheat or escape death by having his head transplanted onto the body of a young adult killed in a car wreck. The moral and ethical dilemmas stemming from these developments become even more challenging, when considering the fact that some bodies might be grown in test tubes.

Recent advances in biotechnology have generated the possibility that scientists soon will be able to grow human organs and body parts on an industrial scale in laboratory conditions. These might range from noses and ears to hearts, lungs and livers.

If such scientific advances continue to progress as some people hope, perhaps scientists will be able to create or clone entire human bodies—grown under laboratory conditions. When and if this happens, would transplanting an elderly person's head onto one of these fresh bodies be considered moral and ethical? Also, on a spiritual level, do our bodies have souls—and, if so, can the essence of us be transferred to another body?

The thing about death is that it's honest.

-Laura Linney

Another issue involving the morality of death is likely to arise with the development of human clones.

Based on technologies developed in recent years, scientists may soon be able to create an exact replica of a naturally conceived human being. Under laboratory conditions, this could be done by taking cells from the person and essentially growing a completely new but identical individual in a test-tube environment.

Would the clones have souls?

Would indiscriminately killing them be considered legal, since those individuals would not be conceived naturally as taught by most religions and spiritual beliefs?

Would the intentional killing of the original donor be considered permissible because that individual has a "mirror image" to replace him?

The number of potential moral and ethical questions could become seemingly endless. While fearing that such technology could eventually develop into "commonplace occurrences," I consider such prospects as repulsive and morally confusing.

A man whose life has been dishonorable is not entitled to escape disgrace in death.
 -Lucius Accius

Chapter 25

Meet the "Grim Reaper"

Particularly since the Middle Ages, death has been considered a repulsive, often-demonic and much-unwanted shadowy figure.

Traditions that continue today in modern European folklore motivate people in many cultures worldwide to call death "The Grim Reaper."

Often coming suddenly and without warning, this character is said to wear a dark cloak or hood while carrying a "scythe"—an agricultural tool for mowing grass or reaping crops. This unwanted character also is sometimes called the Angel of Death or even the Devil of Death, occasionally referred to as the "angel of dark and light."

Some people worry that the Grin Reaper actually can cause death. This in turn has led people to create classic tales in which key characters attempt to bribe this spirit or entity in hopes of extending their own lives.

Various nations and religions ranging from Christians to Jews have all had their own legends or beliefs regarding this entity.

You've got to know what death is to know life!

-Jack Kavorkian

Death and particularly the Grim Reaper have transcended recent and current popular culture. Death has been a recurring character in the Discworld novel series.

James W. Forsythe, M.D., H.M.D.

In a popular 1957 movie chronicling the Crusades, "The Seventh Seal," a character portrayed by Igmar Bergman plays chess with death. Bergman's character strives to win the game in hopes of saving his own life.

The Grim Reaper or similar characters depicting Death have been featured in a variety of TV shows including the "Twilight Zone" from the late 1950s and early 1960s.

More recently, Death has been portrayed a title character in movies, including "Meet Joe Black" and "Death Takes a Holiday."

A frequent character on the current animated TV show "Family Guy," Death when portrayed as the Grim Reaper also has appeared in such films as "Monty Python's the Meaning of Life" in 1983, and "Castlevania" in 2013, appearing as Dracula's assistant.

A toilet-humor animated TV series that appeared on the Cartoon Network from 2003 to 2008, "The Grim Adventures of Billy and Mandy" featured the character "Grim" modeled after death.

Collectively and individually, these various programs and many others featuring the Grim Reaper were designed to generate horror, pure entertainment or laughter. Throughout modern culture depictions of our eventual demise enable us to laugh at or to fear our eventual demise—although we rarely give that outcome much serious thought.

In an artwork you're always looking for artistic decisions, so an ashtray is perfect. An ashtray has got life and death.

-Damien Hirst

Besides the Grim Reaper, most major cultures have developed various uniquely individual characters, each designed to personify death.

These have ranged from the First Lady of the Underworld in the ancient Babylonian society to the Lady of Death, sometimes called the "Queen of Mictlan" in the ancient Aztec culture.

About Death

Besides Hades, the king of the Underworld mentioned much earlier, the Ancient Greek Mythology had many characters all depicting death. These included Thanatos, a spirit of death and mortality, and Erebus, a primeval god of darkness.

Mankind's many other efforts to personify death, and thus attempt to mentally cope with that outcome also ranged from the gods Odin, Hel and Freyja in Greek mythology, to the Roman's Pluto, ruler of the underworld.

The numerous other Death characters that became increasingly popular hundreds or thousands of years ago spread across the Hindu, Eastern Asian and European cultures.

Perhaps one of the most destructive of these spirits was Angra Mainyu, an angel of death or destructive spirit feared by the Ancient Persians.

Death is like an arrow that is already in flight, and your life lasts only until it reaches you.
-Georg Hermes

Since its inception more than 230 years ago, the United States has gradually accepted varying forms of dark humor in which the viewer laughs at morbid depictions of death.

Sometimes called "black comedy" or "adult comedy," today's variations of black comedy generally depict a morbid, dark aura surrounding both life and death.

The term "black humor" was not intended as a form of racism and cultural differences rarely become an issue in such plots. Nonetheless, some individuals might find the use of the term as offensive or problematic.

Accelerating in the mid-1930s at the height of the Great Depression, "black humor" evolved into a subset of the overall comedy category. Ultimately, this genre depicts a skeptical or cynical view of life, essentially signifying that "everything is going to die anyway—so everything in this life is pointless."

James W. Forsythe, M.D., H.M.D.

Naturally and quite predictably, such attempts at humor struck many people as repulsive and offensive, particularly from the view of religious zealots. The frequency of plots that drew sympathy for characters that torment people drew equally intense contempt from some audience members.

Some audiences laughed uproariously, while also simultaneously feeling at least somewhat repulsed.

I am one who believes that one of the greatest dangers of advertising is not that of misleading people, but that of boring them to death.

-Leo Burnett

The overall popularity of black humor transferred from the stage into contemporary literature.

Some of the most popular yet highly controversial writers who frequently employed black humor during the 20th Century included Joseph Heller and John Bart.

Edward Albee's highly controversial play "Whose Afraid of Virginia Woolf" in 1962, a one-act play "The Zoo Story" in 1958, and "The Sandbox" in 1959 had varying degrees of success—while drawing criticism from those repulsed by black humor.

Nonetheless, largely due to his ability to focus directly with fear and death, Albee also drew praise. Other authors who gained notoriety for black comedy included Heller, author of the black comedy "Catch-22," so popular the term was added to dictionaries.

A steady succession of writers gained notoriety and popularity, including Kurt Vonnegut, Phillip Roth, Ronald Dahl, Warren Zevon and Thomas Pynchon Jr.

Far more than ever since its earliest days, the United States evolved into a culture that at least occasionally accepted or laughed at a defeatist attitude toward life and death.

Topics broached frequently by the most famous of these authors included events that some deemed as politically thought

About Death

provoking. With death almost always the overriding ultimate theme, domestic violence, murder and suicide evolved into hot topics.

Often resulting in death or at least "much wanted death," additional plotlines delved into mutilation, drug abuse, terminal illness, disabilities, racism, and homophobia. Much of the time the characters either preferred death to these lifestyles or afflictions, or the factors ultimately resulted in their demise.

The most dire disaster in love is the death of imagination.

-George Meredith

As the popularity of black comedy clicked into fear in the American culture, one of the most successful depictions on film was "Doctor Strangelove" in 1964.

The Stanley Kubrick film, starring Slim Pickens, Peter Sellers and George C. Scott, is still heralded as perhaps one of the most popular movies of its genre; it dealt with nuclear warfare and the annihilation of the earth.

The popular 1970s TV sitcom "M*A*S*H," depicting life in a U.S. military base during the Korean War, brought death and black comedy to American livings like never before. Embracing the long-held pattern of this genre, the program portrayed battle scenes as particularly absurd.

Long before black comedy became "the rage" in America, serious and scary stories of the macabre permeated most cultures worldwide. Most plots in this genre, from books to movies, involve vivid symbols of death or wretched stories about dying.

Since the onset of humanity such tales have gripped the imagination, probably because people have always remained fascinated by death no matter what their particular individual religious beliefs might dictate.

Edgar Allen Poe gained a reputation during the early 1800s, living just to age 40 from 1810 to 1850. Although excelling during the romantic movement in literature, he became prolific at the macabre and mysteries.

Poe's riveting writing skills and boundless imagination enabled him to tap a American fascination with death that had been previously unfulfilled. In 1845, just five years before his death, Poe published his world-famous poem "The Raven." Many of his short "tales" and poems were published in magazines.

One of his most acclaimed short stories, "A Premature Burial" chronicled the fictional tale of what a person endured after being buried in a grave—although not actually having died. Many of his stories remain required reading among high school students, including "The Pit and the Pendulum," about a prisoner tortured during the Spanish Inquisition.

Within the American culture, horror stories and weird fiction steeped in death became popular thanks largely to such authors as H.P. Lovecraft during the 1900s. His writing became so powerful that some critics described him as the Edgar Allen Poe of the 20th Century.

Lovecraft's books inspired numerous successful films including "Call of the Cthulhu: Dark Corners of the Earth," and "id Software's Quake."

I get scared to death when I see people who say they've found Jesus Christ, and they're out there, and I wonder, who's teaching them? Who's mentoring them?

-Willie Aames

The great legendary bard William Shakespeare was perhaps the first playwright to successfully romanticize death, long before the era of Poe and others that followed.

Besides "Romeo & Juliet," previously mentioned, Shakespeare's plots virtually all delved into the topic of death.

Universally and generally considered as perhaps the greatest author of all time, Shakespeare deftly touched on this critical subject that has mystified mankind in everything from "Macbeth" and "Hamlet," to "A Midsummer Night's Dream."

Besides enviable skills for writing and prose, Shakespeare managed to delve deeply into the essence of what almost everyone has feared.

His tales and plotting have transcended the generations, becoming perhaps the first person to deeply infiltrate the topic of death on a widespread scale.

The countless writers that have followed have dwelled on numerous specific genres where death becomes integral. Authors gaining fame in the modern era have included Stephen King specializing in horror and the macabre, and John Grisham, famous for courtroom sagas that often involve death or the threat of murder.

Since time immemorial people have yearned for compelling, heart-stopping tales about death. These permeated into recent and current television, where the likes of Perry Mason played by the late Raymond Burr, airing on CBS-TV from 1957 to 1966, victoriously strived weekly to solve a murder in a courtroom setting. Streams of detective dramas and courtroom sagas evolved into successful TV episodes in the decades that followed.

Just like the poles of a magnet, some people are drawn to death and others are repulsed by it, but we all have to deal with it.
-James Hetfield

Our fascination with death in the American culture remained unsatisfied throughout the last half of the 20th Century. Entertainers in the new music genre of rock 'n' roll often crooned about death starting in the 1950s, a topic that intensified during the heavy metal and punk rock eras of the late 1970s and early 1980s.

Indeed, our culture cannot seem to get enough of death in plots, movies, books and songs, although we individually shun any serious thought or discussion on the topic.

James W. Forsythe, M.D., H.M.D.

The death of the "rock king" Elvis Presley at age 42 in 1977 shocked many people into the realization that death can strike anyone, even world-famous individuals, at relatively early age.

Although the iconic rock star Michael Jackson had gained a reputation for alleged drug abuse, his death at age 50 in 2009 stunned fans worldwide.

Mysteriously, world-renowned legendary figures such as Elvis and Jackson seem to remain "alive" in the public mindset, their separate estates now earning far more annually than during the final years when they were "above ground."

This, in turn, can serve as a symbol or message that each and every one of us today can seem to remain alive—even after we're gone from this earth.

You can't choreograph death, but you can choreograph your funeral.

-Marina Abramovic

Chapter 26

My Own Death

"**D**octor Forsythe, how are you going to die if you're such an expert at the process?" some people might want to ask, now that I have explained most of what's involved.

Well, if you must know, before I die my ongoing process of living life to the fullest will continue unabated for as long as possible.

Now in relatively good health, while now in my mid-70s I continue to expect a long and fruitful life for many years to come.

For me, a fulfilling, whole and complete life embossed with happiness means teaching others while spending quality time with people that I love and truly care about.

Until my dying day, I will continue to write books on essential issues that people care about. Working diligently in a non-stop effort to extend the lives of people with cancer also remains a top priority, while additionally helping a select few highly qualified doctors learn the techniques of natural treatments that have enabled me to help many people.

Why would you be afraid of death? It would be an inconvenience. I have a lot of undone things and it's bound to get in the way. But, no, it doesn't scare me at all.
-David Carradine

As a health care professional with extensive expertise on the life and death process, I realize that my life might end suddenly and without any warning.

Yet my mental attitude shall always remain positive even if my health should suddenly start failing. Remember, as stated earlier, I've witnessed countless instances where people with a winning, can-do mindset have whipped potentially fatal afflictions.

Be that as it may, I also know that even positive attitudes ultimately fail against the Grim Reaper, for Mother Nature dictates that we all must die.

But am I afraid?

Just as important, are you terrified as well if you're not deemed terminally ill, or if you have a close relative or loved one now in the process of dying?

Well, if you ask me, I would say that fear will do none of us any good when facing death. The best "weapon" for helping ourselves and others regarding death is love.

If we openly declare what is wrong with us, what is our deepest need, then perhaps the death and despair will by degrees disappear.

-J.B. Priestly

Until taking my final breath, I shall possess a continual "professional love" for all my patients and staff. My love and caring heart for my wife Earlene, for our children and grandchildren shall last through all eternity.

My message here serves as a blessing. Yes, our Creator has given me the heart, knowledge and passion to bring this message to you here.

The mysterious and intrigue of death becomes insignificant upon our final breaths, while the blessings of our lives can never be taken away. Whether we've done "bad" or "good" while in this life, nothing can possibly remove those experiences.

Perhaps above all, at least to me, the essence of our lives is about learning.

Once again, without trying to sound overly preachy or

About Death

condescending, I can say without any doubt whatsoever is that the most important lesson that we learn involves love.

Everybody thinks I'm at death's door, but I'm not. There's nothing seriously wrong with me, and my heart is in 100-percent working order. Anything else you may hear is a damn lie!

-Bobby Darin

    I've seen this message of love in the eyes of my many patients, many who have subsequently died. Similar expressions have beamed from the eyes of my clinic staff, relatives and friends.

    Surely many of these people have emitted sadness and many tears, usually out of anger, grief, fear or both. Strangely, as I've seen many times, these sensations invariably fade if the person lives long enough, while negative reactions get replaced by love.

    Knowing this, many people also might want to ask, "Then Doctor, what is love anyway—and how can we show it, where and when?"

    The best answer I can give here centers on how we think and behave.

    A simple and brief touch on a dying person's hand can display warmth and caring. With just as much brightness in the face of the coming darkness, terminal people can and do often reach out to touch or hug almost anyone around them.

    When my time comes, and it inevitably will as yours does as well, I will either gently touch other people in appropriate ways with my hands. Or, if my body fails to move, I will mentally send out thoughts conveying a similar bond.

Death's an old joke, but each individual encounters it anew.

-Ivan Turgenev

James W. Forsythe, M.D., H.M.D.

For as long as my mind allows, particularly while on my deathbed, I shall remain as mentally at ease as my senses will allow.

All my thoughts shall remain focused on my love for others, and for those who have touched my life. While my mind remains fully functional, I'll be thinking of patients from long ago and the recent past.

Then, I'll know that a lot of them either have or are undergoing a similar experience.

Throughout history many wise people have indicated that "no matter how many people surround you when your time comes, you always die alone—because only you are doing this at the moment, experiencing your personal end in this life."

Perhaps fear will race through my mind. Yet somehow, deep down, I know that "what will be, will be." At that point I certainly will not be able to change the past or control much if anything of what happens in the future.

All I can leave of any meaning is what I have done, in my professional life and in my personal life as well. My legacy will be my love and my passion for life and for helping others when I have been healthy.

I mean, death is a serious thing, certainly not to be sneezed at.

-Steven Patrick Morrissey

So, what past actions of yours if any do you think about today, particularly if in the process of dying or helping someone you know currently experiencing death?

If you feel as though you haven't accomplished much of any worth, let any potential regrets pass above you as if a wandering bird far away.

Instead, think, like I will as well when my time comes, that at least you've had this experience, this life, and you were unique.

About Death

Certainly none of us is perfect, so accepting that fact can help take you a long way toward accepting your own death.

Fully cognizant of these essential factors, at this point while healthy myself I can only suppose that I will quickly pass through the anger and denial phases that Kübler-Ross, author described. As a physician and as an expert in the death process, I fully realize that denial and anger will do nothing whatsoever to help me.

As for you, on the question of how you should deal with these two issues, I can only say that expressing anger and denial will never do you any good in the long run.

If I ever completely lost my nervousness, I would be frightened half to death.

-Paul Lynde

Perhaps I'll throw dinner plates across my hospital patient room due to pent-up anger. But I doubt that ever would occur because I'm simply not that kind of guy.

More likely, I'll become at least somewhat depressed. Yes, I'm only human, and I'm not going to try to proclaim here that I'm superhuman just because I know about death.

Any sadness that I have likely would come from frustration, for I feel that there remains so much more work and so many more good things I can do here on earth.

Yet I know that any eternal continuation of my life here is not and will not be possible, so all of us here have only a limited time. God willing, my many books and medical research reports can continue to serve as a part of my legacy when I'm gone.

With each passing second on the clock as my death approaches, I'll also realize that any sadness that I might find myself feeling is pointless and overly self-centered. And, hopefully, when your own particularly time comes you will feel the same as well.

As individuals, many with families or loved ones, who remain essentially "alone," the acceptance of "what is" can take us a long way to our own conception of "heaven" or "nirvana."

When death has you by the throat, you don't mince words.

- Friedrich Dürrenmatt

The "Tibetan Book of Living and Dying," a steady seller for many years, indicated that monks for thousands of years have believed that in subsequent lifetimes we evolve into what we were at the exact moment of death.

Age-old teachings indicate that monks devote their entire lives to how they will be mentally at the exact second of taking their final breath.

Monks that embrace the concept of reincarnation believe that if a person is hateful and angry when dying, he or she will be embossed with those characteristics in the afterlife and beyond. Conversely, those who "breath in and breath out sensations of the essence of love" right up to their dying moment are said to have this characteristic as they depart and transition forward from this life.

Of course, I'm not a monk or a Buddhist, but rather a Christian who has never strived to be a preacher in any way. Even so, deep down in my heart I believe that the monks' teaching here makes a lot of sense.

Certainly, we can only ever be is what we "are." At the time of death, hate, anger and excessive fear will get us nowhere for the end will come.

So, knowing this, when your time for death arrives, will you choose to remain hateful, vengeful, vindictive and filled with hate—keenly aware all the while that those emotions or sensations will ultimately never do you or anyone any good whatsoever.

About Death

The line between life and death is determined by what we are willing to do.
                                                                -Bear Grylls

    Instead of feeling angry, regretful or vindictive, my hope is that you will be accepting of your particular situation and filled with nothing but the pure essence of love as you die.

    This would be a fitting end for all people, no matter what has killed us—either disease or wounds from tragedies like car accidents.

    Cognizant of the fact that Death can come suddenly at any moment, let us live our lives in love—which under ideal conditions is strong and never weak.

    Simply live your life today in the best way that you can, whether currently healthy or if your final days seem imminent. As your time approaches, I suggest that you try within the confines of your own mind to forgive those who have wronged you.

    If you're able to do so, you'll set yourself free mentally of any potential need to feel groundless and unproductive hate as your moment to step from this world arrives.

    For my part, I have already begun the ongoing process of forgiveness. I have forgiven the many mainstream doctors nationwide who have wrongly criticized me, complaining that natural treatments are worthless—when in fact those methods often have tremendous value to seriously ill people.

    I also forgive, at least on an emotional level, those federal prosecutors who once filed bogus, trumped-up criminal charges against me. I was ultimately found innocent by a jury of my peers who found that I never committed any wrongdoing when administering a natural substance—human growth hormone—to some patients.

I love myself. Anything that has my name, I'm tickled to death.
                                                                -Barbara Corcoran

James W. Forsythe, M.D., H.M.D.

Healthy while writing and publishing this book, I spent at least some time daily praying for all of my past, current and future patients.

I pray to the Lord, asking that He may grant each and every one of us a peaceful death—grateful and thankful that each and every one of us once have been alive.

When sudden death takes a president, opportunities for new beginning flourish, among the ambitious and the tensions among such people can be dramatic, as they were when President Kennedy was killed.

-Russell Baker

My mother's songs are really turning out to be masterpieces. I have inherited this incredible legacy and am so fortunate to bathe in her sensibilities. It is tinged with tragedy. I'd much rather she was here in person, but there is still a positive force to come out of her death and that is having the gift of music that she gave.

-Rufus Wainwright

The need to understand prescription information can literally be a matter of life and death.

-Andrew Cuomo

About the Author

James W. Forsythe, M.D., H.M.D., has long been considered one of the most respected physicians in the United States, particularly for his treatment of cancer and the legal use of human growth hormone. In the mid-1960s, Dr. Forsythe graduated with honors from University of California at Berkeley and earned his medical degree from the University of California, San Francisco, before spending two years residency in Pathology at Tripler Army Hospital, Honolulu. After a tour of duty in Vietnam, he returned to San Francisco and completed an internal medicine residency and an oncology fellowship. He is also a world-renowned speaker and author. He has co-authored, been mentioned in and/or written in numerous bestselling or hot-selling books. To name a few: "An Alternative Medicine Definitive Guide to Cancer;" "Knockout, Interviews with Doctors who are Curing Cancer," Suzanne Somers' number one bestseller; "The Ultimate Guide to Natural Health, Quick Reference A-Z Directory of Natural Remedies for Diseases and Ailments;" "Anti-Aging Cures;" "The Healing Power of Sleep;" "Anti-Aging Sleep Secrets;" "Outsmart Your Cancer: Alternative Non-Toxic Treatments That Work;" and "Compassionate Oncology—What Conventional Cancer Specialists Don't Want You To Know;" and "Obaminable Care," "Complete Pain;" "Natural Painkillers;" and "Your Secret to the Fountain of Youth—What They Don't Want You to Know About HGH Human Growth Hormone;" "Take Control of Your Cancer;" and the "Emergency Radiation Medical Handbook."

Contact Information
Century Wellness Clinic, 521 Hammill Lane
Reno, NV, 89511
(775) 827-0707
RenoWellnessDr@Yahoo.com